Contents

4

Preface

IEA *Research Monographs* accommodate texts in which the emphasis is normally on the empirical content derived from documentary evidence, field studies, or other sources.

Research Monograph 40, *Which Doctor?*, is a study of professional restrictive practices in Britain's monopoly National Health Service. Its author, Dr David Green, is not a medical doctor but a political scientist and an historian of the welfare state.[1] This *Monograph* has arisen out of his investigations into the supply of health care prior to the establishment of the NHS in 1948. His research has shown that between the wars medical care was provided to the uninsured (which in the late-1930s amounted to just under half of the population—mainly women and children) by a variety of competing sources and that the presence of competition worked to restrain medical fees. Most notable among the organisations in that competitive market were the friendly society medical institutes and a number of Welsh works clubs (medical aid societies).

In an Historical Postscript to this *Monograph*, the author gives a blow-by-blow account of how the medical institutes and medical aid societies—which had not only helped to contain the price of medical treatment but had also pioneered new services—were killed off by political action in order to leave the field clear for the NHS monolith. Central to that story is the decisive pressure which the British Medical Association as the doctors' trade union brought upon the politicians to sign the death warrant. The institutes and societies had attracted the deep hostility of the BMA because their competitive activities made it difficult for the BMA to organise doctors in an effective cartel. If government could be persuaded to remove the competition—and the establishment of the NHS provided an occasion not to be missed—a thousand restrictive practices could bloom.

---

[1] Among his published works is IEA Occasional Paper 63, *The Welfare State: For Rich or for Poor?* (1982).

As the author documents, the medical profession had already in the first half of this century become increasingly adept both at inducing government to narrow the field of competition and at 'capturing' the agency that was supposed to regulate it, namely, the General Medical Council. With the advent of the NHS monopoly, the doctors' cartel was well entrenched to advance its members' interests at the expense of the consumer (and the taxpayer).

In the principal part of his *Monograph*, Dr Green applies the lessons he draws from this historical episode to rebut the argument that the most effective way to improve health care in Britain would be to reform the NHS—through such devices as training in better management skills, new incentive mechanisms, and tighter budgetary controls. In his view, improvement is conditional on eliminating the state-imposed barriers to competition in the supply of health care. Without competition—and especially competition among doctors—cartelised professional resistance within the NHS will continue to stymie structural and managerial reforms.

Dr Green takes particular issue with what he calls 'supply-side' advocates of the NHS—or the 'York school', since three leading exponents hold chairs at the University of York. According to the author, supply-siders, while frequently very critical of the NHS as it now is and impatient to reform it, nonetheless remain committed to the ideals of the NHS because of its potential to control the professionals whom they regard as enjoying far too much power. They thus prize the NHS as a countervailing force to the organised medical profession. Moreover, they maintain, the market cannot work in health care for two additional reasons: first, because the knowledge of the doctor is so superior to that of the patient that ordinary consumer choice is not feasible; and, secondly, because third-party financing of health care offers no incentives to doctors or patients to behave in a cost-effective way. Since, it is claimed, these problems are common to both the NHS and the market, more of the market will not improve health care; the best hope is to reform the NHS.

Dr Green argues that the supply-siders are mistaken in believing consumer sovereignty is impossible in health care and so concluding that the market has little to contribute. The York school's solution to the consumer's vulnerability to the unscrupulous doctor is, he suggests, to put the former even more at the mercy of the latter through the NHS. He reproves the supply-siders on four principal grounds. First, they wrongly equate the market in health care with the system in the USA which is only *in part* the product of the market and whose defects are due not to market failure but to unwise state intervention. Secondly, they assume the market failed historically in Britain, whereas the evidence is that prior to the NHS the market devised mechanisms for maintaining efficiency and providing good, low-cost service. Thirdly, the supply-siders fail to take sufficient account of the theory of public choice[1] which would predict that the self-interested power of doctors will not easily be curtailed in a state monopoly industry. And, fourthly, supply-siders ignore the neo-Austrian insight that a competitive market is not merely a mechanism for economising but also, in Hayek's famous phrase, a 'discovery procedure'.

After a lengthy analysis of specific restrictive practices in the medical profession, Dr Green concludes that the power of doctors derives largely from legal privileges and immunities unwisely granted them *by the state*. In his view, neither the NHS nor the market can produce more cost-effective health care without a radical and direct assault on those privileges and immunities. Unfortunately for the supply-siders, however, the NHS is itself a major institutional buttress to the power of the organised medical profession.

Undaunted, Dr Green offers 10 policy proposals to curb restrictive practices in the profession and inject a whiff of competition into the activities of doctors. Essentially, his proposals entail removing the profession's immunities from the general law and replacing the General Medical Council with a new regulatory agency whose powers would be confined to protecting the consumer and whose constitution would safeguard it from 'capture' by the profession.

Although the Institute is obliged to dissociate its Trustees, Directors and Advisers from the analysis and conclusions of this *Research Monograph*, it offers Dr Green's study as a fascinating glimpse into the world of restrictive practices in the professions. Despite the Government's recent well-publicised tussles with the opticians and the solicitors, it remains something of a closed world, ripe for further disinterested exploration. Dr Green has beaten a fertile path for others to follow.

July 1985   Martin Wassell

---

[1] An introduction to the theory of public choice is provided by Gordon Tullock in *The Vote Motive*, Hobart Paperback 9, IEA, 1976, and by James M. Buchanan *et al.* in *The Economics of Politics*, IEA Readings 18, IEA, 1978.

Author's Introduction

This *Research Monograph* originated in a study of the friendly societies and general practitioner services before the National Health Service (NHS). The findings are to be published by Maurice Temple Smith under the title *Working Class Patients and the Medical Establishment*. This paper extends the historical analysis a little further and discusses the obstacles which stand in the way of reforming the NHS. Those obstacles form a barrier not only against public policy-makers who wish to retain the NHS structure in all essentials whilst improving its cost-effectiveness; they stand equally in the path of analysts who advocate much more consumer sovereignty in health care. This *Monograph* analyses the emerging supply-side case for the NHS now being advanced and proposes an alternative, libertarian strategy of reform.

The 'Historical Postscript' explores a little-known series of events in the emergence of the NHS. The episode described is of interest for two reasons. It reveals how the government's wish to please the British Medical Association (BMA) led to the suppression of the remaining element of choice available to the consumer; and it provides an apt illustration of what Hayek has called the 'synoptic delusion'. Orthodox economists are accustomed to thinking of the market as a mechanism for the allocation of resources between sectors. As Hayek and his Austrian school colleagues have shown, however, this interpretation is based on a misunderstanding of what the market can achieve. It is, above all, a procedure for discovering new ways of meeting human wants. This view is so little understood that I have felt it necessary to devote special attention to supporting it. The 'Historical Post-script' shows how, in 1948, the NHS swept aside the last remnants of competition in health care on the assumption that the acknowledged pioneering efforts of the private sector would no longer be required. The importance of leaving room for innovation and experiment was neither understood nor anticipated.

The panel system, established in 1913, significantly reduced competition in the supply of medical care. But one remnant of the vigorous competition of the pre-1913 period remained within the state medical service. There was provision for 'approved institutions' to register under the 1911 National Insurance Act. These were the medical aid societies of the Welsh miners and the medical institutes of the English friendly societies. The 'Historical Postscript' describes how these organisations met their fate when the NHS was being founded, and analyses the reasons for their demise.

June 1985   David G. Green

The Author

DAVID G GREEN was born in Norfolk and educated at the University of Newcastle upon Tyne, 1970-73, where he studied Political
Science and Sociology. He undertook postgraduate research at
the same university, which awarded him a doctorate in 1980.
Whilst a postgraduate he lectured part-time at Newcastle upon
Tyne Polytechnic. From 1972 until 1981 he was a Labour Party
activist, serving as a Labour councillor on Newcastle city council
from 1975 to 1981. He held office as chairman or vice-chairman
of a number of committees or sub-committees, and served as a
governor of three schools. He is currently a Research Fellow at
the IEA, having until recently been a Research Fellow at the
Australian National University.

Dr Green is the author of three books: *Power and Party in an
English City* (London: Allen & Unwin, 1981); (with L. Cromwell)
Mutual Aid or Welfare State: Australia's Friendly Societies (Sydney:
Allen & Unwin, 1984); and *Working Class Patients and the Medical
Establishment*: *Self-Help in Britain From the Mid-Nineteenth
Century to 1948* (London: Temple Smith, forthcoming). The IEA
has previously published his *The Welfare State: For Rich or for
Poor?* (Occasional Paper 63, 1982). His work has also been pub-
lished in journals such as *Municipal Review, The Journal of Social
Policy, Political Quarterly, Public Administration, Philosophy of
the Social Sciences*, and *Economic Affairs*.

He is currently working on a textbook guide to the 'New Right',
commissioned by Wheatsheaf Books.

Acknowledgements

First, I must thank Arthur Seldon for his extremely valuable criticisms of an early draft of this *Research Monograph*. I am also grateful to Hugh Elwell for discussing with me the 'political realism' of the proposals, and to Professor Robert Pinker for his helpful 'friendly-hostile' criticism. Finally, I have to express my appreciation to Michael Solly and Martin Wassell of the IEA's editorial staff.

June 1985   D.G.G.

ONE

The Supply-Side Advantages of the NHS

For most of the life of the NHS, demand-side arguments have been used to justify its existence: the NHS was vital to ensure that the poor did not go without health care, or to guarantee 'equal' access to the best medical care available, or to bring about allocation according to 'need'. In recent years the justification has begun to change. Increasingly, the NHS is being supported because it is believed to offer advantages on the supply side. In the view of Professor A. J. Culyer, for instance, the real argument for the NHS structure lies in its potential to control the professionals who, he believes, enjoy too much power. It could monitor their performance in the light of 'socially, not merely medically, determined objectives'.[1]

Supply-siders' criticism of but commitment to the NHS

Compared with the traditional demand-side advocates of the NHS, supply-siders like Culyer and his colleagues at the University of York, Professors Alan Maynard and Alan Williams, are more willing to admit the faults of the NHS. Indeed, they are scathing in their criticism of partisans who idealise the NHS. However, they remain committed to the *ideals* of the National Health Service.[2] They also believe that, compared with the NHS, the market has little to commend it. A recent study of the public and private sectors in health care carried out by Professor Maynard and Gordon McLachlan concluded:

'This book shows that whatever the public/private mix, be it the 50/50 role of the State and the market in the USA, the 98/2 role of the State and the market in the UK, or any (e.g. Dutch) alternative between these roles,

---

[1] A. J. Culyer [1976], p. 147. [Most of the footnote references to sources in this *Research Monograph* are given in this abbreviated form. The full source reference can be found in the 'List of References' starting on page 78.—ED.]

[2] For example, A. Maynard and A. Williams [1984], p. 110.

partnership between public and private producers is inevitable but the need of cost control is a dominant factor and regulation to achieve universal goals is ubiquitous and inevitable . . . Shifting the public/private mix does not remove regulations; it has a marginal effect and in reality merely changes its nature . . .'[1]

Such regulation, they say, is unavoidable because of the inherent nature of the health-care market:

'monopolies fix the prices, quantities, and qualities of the goods and services they sell in a manner advantageous to them (the providers) rather than the clients (patients); social institutions (the NHS and insurance companies, both private and social) reduce the price barriers to consumption and provide incentives for patients to over-consume (moral hazard) because a third party (the taxpayer or the insurance contributor) pays; and there are few incentives for decision-makers (doctors and managers of various sorts) to behave efficiently (i.e. to ensure costs are minimised and benefit maximised)'.[2]

Professor Maynard even goes so far as to suggest that health-care problems are the same in public or private systems, 'wherever you go on this planet'.[3] The conclusion he draws is that we should focus our efforts on improving the NHS and not on extending the private sector.

Does the analysis of the York school—as I will call Maynard, Culyer, Williams, *et al.*—represent a valid view of the market? I will argue that their analysis is based on a decisive flaw, namely, that they have attributed all the faults of health-care systems containing any kind of market element to the market as such. The passage quoted above indicates how they have gone wrong. They are aware that the 'market' they draw on most for illustration, health care in the USA, is a 50/50 public/private health-care system. In other words, it is not a *pure* market system. They are also aware that many other systems are mixed. But they fail to draw the self-evident conclusion that the attribution of cause and effect is consequently not straightforward. It certainly cannot be assumed that whatever problems exist in *mixed* systems are all due entirely to the defects of the market. This would be to ignore the possibility that the actions of government may be at the root of a problem, or may have exacerbated it.

Government intervention and 'market failures'

Mixed systems produce outcomes which are the product of

---

[1] G. McLachlan and Maynard [1982], pp. 553-54.

[2] *Ibid.*; also Maynard [1982], p. 508.

[3] Maynard [1982], p. 472.

government intervention as well as of the tendencies of the market. To understand fully how a particular situation came about it is vital, therefore, to try to disentangle those outcomes produced by government action from those produced by the market.

The York school identifies three main, universal defects in the supply of health care:

1. Consumer ignorance which results in professional dominance.

2. Third-party funding (private or government) offers no incentives to doctors or patients to behave in a cost-effective manner.

3. Professional (monopoly) power of doctors.

Other 'market failures' are also identified, notably externalities and the inability of the market to supply public goods. These are not, however, central to the supply-side analysis of the York school with which this *Research Monograph* is concerned.[1]

---

[1] The 'caring externality' case for the NHS is argued by Culyer [1976].

TWO

The Doctor/Patient Information Asymmetry

The doctor is believed to have so much knowledge compared with the patient that ordinary consumer choice cannot operate. The doctor is the patient's agent, not only *supplying* medical care but also deciding the quantity and type of care to be *demanded*. According to the York school, this is so in both the market and the NHS: in the market the doctor 'mediates demand on behalf of consumers', and in the NHS he 'identifies the patient's needs'.[1] Because the consumer faces the same difficulty in both the market and the NHS, the York school reasons that the extension of the market will make no difference, and that public policy-makers should therefore focus on overcoming the problem within the NHS. A reformed NHS, Yorkists contend, could best combine the aim of improving the quality of medical care with the goal of minimising costs. Consumer sovereignty can accomplish this end in the production of many goods and services, but in health care it cannot.

Their argument is an improvement on earlier discussions of the agency relationship, which tended to regard the NHS as unproblematically superior to the market. The York school believes that the NHS in its present form is no better than the market. Priorities are not, in reality, determined by patients' needs, but by 'the doctor's own professional situation, by his assessment of the patient's condition, and the expected trouble-making proclivities of the patient'.[2] Other analysts who draw attention to the ignorance of the consumer, such as Professor Brian Abel-Smith, appear to prefer the NHS—even as it now stands—to the market. In Abel-Smith's view, there are 'few fields of consumer expenditure where the consumer is as ill-equipped to exercise his theoretical sovereignty as in health services'.[3]

---

[1] Maynard and Williams [1984], pp. 104-5.
[2] *Ibid.*
[3] B. Abel-Smith [1976], p. 48.

Putting the consumer at the producer's mercy

The York school's solution to the vulnerability of the consumer to the unscrupulous doctor is paradoxically to put the consumer even more at the mercy of the producer through the NHS. They deserve credit for recognising that the NHS, as it stands, offers no solution to the agency relationship. I shall argue, however, that they are mistaken in regarding consumer sovereignty in health care as an impossibility, and in concluding that the market has consequently little to contribute.

The York school is not much concerned to increase patients' choice: the desirable outcome is cost-effective health care. 'Choice' has no real place in its thinking, presumably because Yorkists believe the consumer to be ill-equipped to exercise it. In this respect the York school must be distinguished from those proponents of the NHS who (like Yorkists) favour NHS ideals and want to see reform, but who also want to see choice extended. Advocates of choice within the NHS are usually politicians trying to respond to public opinion without damaging the system too much. As Professor Rudolf Klein has cogently argued, the guiding principle of the NHS is that health care should be 'provided according to need, not in response to demand'. He goes on:

'. . . indeed, it can be argued that the real achievement of the NHS is to *minimise* the total expenditure on health care, while making rationing— which may, in some circumstances even mean turning away to die people who could be helped . . . —socially and politically acceptable'.[1]

'Choice' is popular, but choice means health care based on demand and not allocated according to 'need'. Thus NHS partisans who say they want choice are faced with wanting two incompatible things.

The Royal Commission on the NHS (RCNHS) of 1979 exemplified this attitude of being both for and against choice. It considered maximum freedom of choice to be desirable. Doctors should explain the options and wherever possible leave the patient to choose. The patient should be free to choose whether to consult a doctor, to change his doctor, to choose a hospital or unit (with a GP's help), or to refuse treatment (except when others are endangered). But the Commission's Report added:

'It is misleading to pretend that the NHS can meet all expectations. Hard choices have to be made. It is a prime duty of those concerned in the provision of health care to make it clear to the rest of us what we can reasonably expect'.[2]

---

[1] Rudolf Klein [1982], p. 101.   [2] RCNHS [1979], p. 11.

This assertion begs a number of questions, but above all assumes that it is for the experts to tell us what we can reasonably expect. To the liberal and the libertarian this is nonsense. It is not the government's business to dictate what any person can 'reasonably expect'. Nor is it the doctor's business. It is for each person to decide, in the light of the best information available, how much cash he wishes to allocate to health—and for doctors to respond accordingly.

Does consumer ignorance render the market unworkable?

I return now to the York school's attitude to the imbalance in knowledge between doctor and patient. Whilst recognising that the problem affects both market systems and the NHS, they make two questionable assumptions: first, they implicitly assume that markets and the NHS face the problem to a broadly equal extent; and, secondly, they assume that there is a better chance of reforming the NHS than of reforming the market to overcome the imbalance.

Is it valid to assume that the market is unworkable because of the asymmetry between the information at the disposal, respectively, of the doctor and the patient? Have all medical markets failed for this reason? We know that, historically, devices emerged in the medical market in this country to speed up the information flow to patients and to enable checks to be placed on doctors.[1]

The reason why the York school regards the market as universally unable to cope with the supply of health care is that evidence from the USA suggests doctors there are able to 'create' demand, particularly for surgery. This is connected with the fee-for-service method of charging. A number of scholars have argued from American or Canadian evidence that, because of the doctor's superior knowledge, supply is the most important determinant of demand.[2] V. R. Fuchs has quantified the relationship: a 10 per cent increase in surgeons, he estimates, leads to a 3 per cent increase in operations.[3] In an older study, M. S. Feldstein contends that the agency relationship enables doctors to exercise similar power within the zero-priced NHS.[4]

---

[1] Green [1984] and *Working Class Patients and the Medical Establishment* [forthcoming].

[2] A. S. Detsky [1978], pp. 38-9, 139-46; R. G. Evans [1974].

[3] V. R. Fuchs [1978], pp. 35-36.

[4] M. S. Feldstein [1967], pp. 196-200, 278-80.

Other studies, however, contradict this view. F. A. Sloan and R. Feldman, for example, maintain that some economists have been 'much too hasty' in concluding that supply is a 'major demand determinant'.[1] They argue that, for consumer demand to count in the market-place, it is not necessary for *all* consumers to be perfectly informed, or even well informed. It is necessary only that *some* consumers are able to assess the service being offered *and* are willing to seek out lower prices. Without in any way implying that cameras are like health care in *every* respect, Sloan and Feldman cite Mark Pauly's assertion:

> 'I know even less about the works of a movie camera than I know about my own organs; yet I feel fairly confident in purchasing a camera for a given price as long as I know that there are at least a few experts in the market who are keeping sellers reasonably honest'.[2]

J. P. Newhouse, A. P. Williams *et al.* have shown[3] that, as their numbers have grown, specialist doctors have increasingly had to move out of larger towns—even though they preferred to live there—because they could not create sufficient demand. J. Hadley, J. Holahan and W. Scanlon found that, after the introduction of Medicare in Canada, real medical incomes fell. Fees were under strict control and prices for supplies, office space, secretarial help, and so on rose to produce an erosion of medical incomes.[4] From this and Californian evidence, the authors conclude that doctors do have the ability to create demand but that it is limited. If the medical profession had an unlimited capacity to create demand for its services, it would not have permitted a real fall in its incomes.

Moreover, many insurance companies have tackled the 'over-consumption' problem by introducing co-insurance, under which the patient pays a proportion of all bills. Evidence from a Rand Corporation study, led by Newhouse, casts serious doubt on the extreme version of the supply-creates-demand thesis: that physicians can offset any changes in demand that might be induced by changes in insurance or other variables. The interim report of the Rand study concluded that 'Cost sharing unambiguously reduces expenditure'.[5]

---

[1] F. A. Sloan and R. Feldman [1978], p. 118.

[2] *Ibid.*, p. 61.

[3] Newhouse, Williams *et al.* [1979].

[4] Hadley, Holahan and Scanlon [1979], pp. 247-58.

[5] Newhouse *et al.* [1982], p. v.; Newhouse [1981], pp. 93-4.

Defects of US health care the result of unwise government intervention

More important, however, is that much of the 'over-consumption' of health care in the USA is not due exclusively to the inherent properties of the market. A number of factors explain the sky-rocketting costs of American health care. And they are the result, in whole or in part, directly or indirectly, of unwise government intervention. The US medical profession has sought to limit competition by enforcing restrictive practices and imposing entry restrictions. Instead of outlawing such devices, governments (mainly state governments) have either permitted their own powers to be put at the disposal of the organised profession or have granted it immunities from general laws governing restrictive practices.[1] Government subsidisation of fee-based medical care for the elderly and the poor, through Medicare and Medicaid, has had a particularly inflationary effect on prices. And government tax relief for employers who offer their staff health insurance programmes has tended to weaken normal incentives to economise in this huge sector of the market. Employers can deduct from tax all their expenditures on health insurance for their workforce; and all benefits received by employees count as non-taxable income. Moves to open up employee groups to more cost-conscious health maintenance organisations (HMOs)[2] in competition with conventional third-party reimbursement plans proved ineffective due to the imposition of an unwieldy official registration process. And legislative efforts to enable Medicare beneficiaries to benefit from HMOs proved a dead letter because the procedure for paying HMOs imposed an implicit tax on them.[3]

The error of the York school is to equate the potentialities of the market with the system in the USA, even though that system is only *in part* the product of the market. Yorkists speak of the US system and the NHS as though they were opposites. Thus they find it paradoxical that the American market and the NHS face apparently similar problems. It is true that the American system exhibits more of the features of a market than does the NHS. But the defects of American health care are due, not to market failure, but to unwise state intervention. The faults of the (state-run) NHS and the American health market therefore have a common root: imprudent state interference. The Yorkist conclusion that (because the American system is defective) an extension of the market

---

[1] Milton Friedman [1962]; R. A. Kessel [1958]; J. L. Berlant [1975].

[2] HMOs are discussed more fully below, pp. 29-30.

[3] A. C. Enthoven [1978], p. 652.

22

would not help to improve British health care is, therefore, logically invalid. Producer power in the USA is, in very large measure, the product of government interference. Yet, even with the huge distortions government actions have produced in the USA, variations in the price of medical care have a significant effect on demand. A reasonable inference from this is that it may be possible to reform the market to enable it to function more efficiently.

THREE

The Missing Incentives to Economise

In the view of the York school, third-party funding agencies, whether private insurance funds or government departments, eliminate incentives to economise and therefore tend to encourage 'over-consumption'. This tendency is reinforced by professional power. According to Maynard, in both the market and the NHS, clinical freedom and professional power have 'led to a failure to create mechanisms which ensure that practitioners evaluate clinical outcomes and their cost implications'. He finds this both inefficient and unethical.[1] In an earlier work, [2] Maynard and Anne Ludbrook propose some devices for improving the cost-effectiveness of the NHS:

> 'The efficiency arguments for the market run aground on the problems of professional monopoly power and the fact that the doctors as a group have behaved in market and NHS bureaucracy environments in the same way: they have failed to evaluate their practices and ensure that society's scarce resources are used efficiently. They have chosen to use practices which are sometimes inefficient, sometimes useless, and sometimes harmful because of their unwillingness to evaluate scientifically their behaviour. As a group, but with noble individual exceptions, they have behaved inefficiently and unethically in both State and private health care systems'.[3]

The market, they argue, will only better the performance of the NHS if it 'generates pressures which force the doctors to evaluate their practices and use resources more efficiently'. But, they conclude, 'such pressure could also be generated by NHS bureaucrats'.

They propose half-a-dozen specific measures. The first priority is improved training, particularly in management skills and health economics. New incentive mechanisms should be introduced, some of which would rely on 'moral suasion', like medical audit;

---

[1] Maynard [1982], p. 487.

[2] Maynard and Ludbrook [1980], pp. 27-41.

[3] *Ibid.*, pp. 32-3.

others would count on the 'sticks-and-carrots' of monetary and non-monetary pressures—filling in special forms, cutting salaries for non-performance and *vice-versa*. Also essential is budget reform so that decision-makers become budget-holders as well. There might also be a role for a health-care inspectorate modelled on the schools inspectorate.[1]

The approach of the York school is certainly an advance on previous justifications for maintaining the NHS. But, as with consumer ignorance, they have misunderstood the true potential of the market mechanism. Yorkists assume (not without some justification) that consumers want cost-effectiveness. They also assume (with far less justification) that this can be accomplished without normal market incentives to economise: in a functioning market it pays the consumer to shop around for low-cost, high-quality health care because he or she can spend the money saved on other valued items; and it pays the producer to keep prices low because failure to do so would mean going out of business.

Members of the York school believe the market cannot help because they assume it failed historically. But the market did devise mechanisms for maintaining efficiency (in the sense of good-standard, low-cost service), as my study of the pre-NHS market shows.[2] And in other health-care systems, market disciplines in operation today (in HMOs, for instance), which are gradually being refined, do serve to encourage better performance. The first task of government should not be the introduction of new and detailed interferences with the clinical freedom of doctors, but to put right the harmful results of its own misguided interference. Above all, reforms should be introduced to modify those aspects of government policy which give the organised profession the whip-hand.

Public choice theory neglected

I turn to these mechanisms below. First, however, there are some wider questions to consider. The York school sees the market as a device for achieving efficient (cost-effective) production. Yet its members note that in the USA (which is closer to being a market than Britain) there are few pressures encouraging cost-effective provision of health care. And they note that there are also few such incentives within the NHS. They therefore mis-

[1] *Ibid.*, pp. 33-5.

[2] David G. Green [1984 and forthcoming].

takenly conclude that the market is incapable of generating cost-effective health care, and that the NHS as it stands is *equally* incapable. But they believe there is a better chance of reforming the NHS than there is of reforming the market.

Their analysis is defective in two respects. First, it fails to take sufficient account of the theory of public choice. Professor Gordon Tullock, a founder of the public-choice school, is critical of traditional economics for employing a 'benevolent despot' model of the political order. He prefers to analyse government as an apparatus, like the market, in which actors try to achieve their private ends. Public choice theory assumes that all individuals in government 'serve their own interests within certain institutional limits'.[1] The difference between government and the market is that 'the limitations within which the individual operates differ'. And, in Tullock's view, the constraints put upon individual conduct in the market are more 'efficient' than those in government. By 'efficient' he means that 'individuals in the market are more likely to serve someone else's well-being when they seek to serve their own than they are in government'.[2] This analysis suggests that the York school may be too optimistic about the prospects for manipulating the NHS environment to achieve cost-effectiveness. The self-interest of doctors will not easily be overcome in *any* predominantly state environment.

The market as a discovery procedure

The second, and more important, defect of the York analysis is that it takes insufficient account of neo-Austrian insights into the true worth of a competitive market. It is not a mere mechanism for economising; it is also, in Professor F. A. Hayek's terminology, a 'discovery procedure'.[3] This function is of vital importance because of the unavoidably dispersed nature of useful knowledge. Professor Maynard's 'sticks-and-carrots' approach presupposes that we know *in advance* which methods of health-care delivery will prove to be the most cost-effective. Government sticks and carrots must be aimed at concrete ends determined in advance. All such specific incentives presume foreknowledge. But in the real world we have no such advance information. It remains to be discovered who will turn out to be the most skilled at remedying particular complaints; who will hit upon the most efficacious

---

[1] Tullock [1976], p. 2.

[2] *Ibid.*, pp. 7, 27.

[3] Hayek [1978], pp. 179-90.

combinations of medication, surgery and after-care; which methods will prove most cost-effective; and which practitioners will prove more able than their colleagues at combining good-quality care with low costs. These are matters which are always in flux and *cannot* be discovered in advance. They cannot, therefore, be built into a state structure such as the NHS.

In practice, applying government sticks and carrots will channel efforts into either compliance or defiance, or some variant in between. Government cannot know which in advance. And, more importantly, state intervention will tend to place a limit on the skill, knowledge and endeavour going into the delivery of health care. In a market, or 'catallaxy' as Hayek prefers,[1] the knowledge that gets used is the knowledge of *all* its members, not merely that held by the central directorate. In a Yorkist health-care scheme, the actors would go about their affairs under constraints intended to channel their efforts in directions dictated by the central power: less knowledge, less skill, and less ingenuity will therefore be brought into play. In a market, with a suitable framework of laws, a bigger array of knowledge and skill is directed at discovering the most cost-effective methods of health-care supply.[2] Instead of having their energies either pent up by government regulations or depleted in efforts to circumvent unwise government rules, those individuals most inclined to innovate and adapt will find themselves better able to do so.

We should therefore aim not at creating sticks and carrots intended to achieve a preordained end-result, but at creating circumstances which make it more likely that most providers of health care will be induced to apply their talents to serving the consumer, including the development of cost-effective methods. In other words, we should aim to create a market.

Three arguments for the market solution

This conclusion may strike some people as implausible. I offer three kinds of argument in support of it: logical, factual, and moral. The first is the logical one. Belief in the value of central direction entails the notion that some decision-maker can be aware of the future state of our knowledge. This is incorrect. The course of human history is strongly influenced by the growth of human knowledge. As Sir Karl Popper has observed: 'if there is such a thing as growing human knowledge, then we cannot

---

[1] Hayek [1973], pp. 14-15; and Hayek [1968].
[2] Hayek [1978], *loc. cit.*

anticipate today what we shall know only tomorrow'.[1] It follows that we cannot predict future developments to the extent that they may be influenced by the growth of knowledge. This problem cannot be entirely overcome, but the market—that is, voluntary co-operation—can reduce the harm that our lack of knowledge of the future may cause. Because our predictions are unreliable, we need to be able to adjust rapidly to unforeseen situations. Voluntary co-operation permits much more flexibility than the coercive machinery of government.

The second argument is that the factual evidence supports the conclusion that the market can supply more cost-effective health care than the NHS. Efforts to put NHS doctors under particular constraints, or to offer incentives intended to channel their efforts in a planned direction, will often be ineffective (if they are not counter-productive) because the decision-maker who devises the incentive (or penalty) does not, and *cannot*, possess the knowledge of all doctors who will be affected. A recent proposal by the Minister of Health to withdraw a number of laxatives from use in the NHS illustrates this limitation. Many patients who take strong painkillers, including cancer victims and some elderly patients, experience regular constipation as a side-effect. This condition causes severe discomfort and in extreme cases can cause death. In the judgement of many doctors the government proposal would have prohibited NHS use of the laxatives most suited to treating such patients. The specific proposal eventually had to be withdrawn in the face of vigorous protests. The Government's strategy of enforcing a limited drugs list, however, continues to be likely to produce unintended effects.[2] A number of products to relieve indigestion, costing around 50 pence, have been prohibited. Doctors who are not willing to displease their patients have available to them on the NHS list only very expensive alternatives intended for other uses. For instance, Tagamet, which costs £16 a course, is normally used to treat stomach ulcers but has recently been advertised as a remedy for 'persistent acid-related' dyspepsia. Ordinarily, a simple antacid would suffice; but a doctor unable to prescribe a suitable antacid under the NHS may well turn to the vastly more expensive Tagamet.[3] Thus, a policy aimed at cutting costs may produce the opposite effect.

West German experience of a similar scheme introduced in 1983

---

[1] Popper [1961], p. x.

[2] This judgement is shared by W. Duncan Reekie, *Competition and Home Medicines*, Research Monograph 39, IEA, May 1985.

[3] *The Times*, 11 February 1985.

bears out this conclusion. Doctors reacted to the blacklisting of some remedies for colds and influenza by prescribing more potent products. This was justified by diagnosing mild conditions as more serious ones. This process, called 'diagnostic drift', resulted in 27 per cent fewer cases of uncomplicated bronchitis being diagnosed whilst diagnoses of chronic bronchitis increased by 21 per cent and acute bronchitis by 61 per cent.[1]

HMOs and the freedom to exit

One of the most cost-effective types of health-care provision is the health maintenance organisation (HMO)—which emerged in the American health market, not in the NHS. Doctors own or contract with the enterprise and patients pay a flat-rate, periodic contribution for all the health care they require during a given period. This financing method encourages a consistent and continuous effort by doctors to treat patients in a cost-effective manner. The evidence is that HMOs offer quality care at lower cost than fee-for-service alternatives. Professor Maynard favours the adaptation of the HMO to NHS conditions by making doctors the local NHS fundholders. (Professor Marshall Marinker has proposed a similar reform,[2] and health Ministers in the Department of Health have shown interest in turning doctors into budget-holders.[3])

We know about HMOs only because it was possible for them to emerge in the American *market-place*. Under a monolithic state system, the emergence of new organisational forms is limited to the range of possibilities that occurs to (or meets with the approval of) the central decision-makers. Evidence from this country supports this conclusion. The nearest service to an HMO in Britain today forms part of Britain's small private sector. The Harrow Health Care Centre is run privately and quite independently of NHS support.[4] Moreover, before the NHS was founded there were organisations with strong resemblances to HMOs—namely, the friendly society medical institutes and the Welsh medical aid societies. They were, however, deliberately put out of business by the state in 1948.[5]

Moreover, HMOs in the USA must satisfy the consumer or go

---

[1] Tony Smith, 'Limited lists of drugs: lessons from abroad', *British Medical Journal*, 16 February 1985, pp. 532-4.

[2] Marinker [1984].

[3] *The Times*, 17 January 1985.

[4] 'Who's afraid of a medical experiment?', *The Economist*, 30 March 1985, pp. 35-6.

[5] 'Historical Postscript', below, pp. 59-77.

broke; this sanction is vital to their success. It is difficult, however, to see how this mechanism could be replicated within a state scheme which refuses to allow patients to determine how to spend their own cash. An end to tax-funding with delivery-in-kind would be a necessary pre-condition for such normal market incentives to be able to emerge. (Because the grip of orthodox opinion is so strong, I have devoted a separate 'Historical Postscript' to showing how the potential for innovation—for 'discovery'—has been stifled by the NHS.)

Coercion morally objectionable

The third argument for a market in health-care supply is a moral one. For the libertarian there are objections of principle to the adoption of a 'sticks-and-carrots' approach by governments. Liberal respect for each individual—doctor and patient alike— demands the minimum of compulsion, and then only to the extent necessary to preserve the common freedoms of all. A free society permits individuals to create and maintain any kind of organisation which seems fitting to them. To deny individuals such freedom is to prevent them from using the detailed knowledge which only they possess and on which alone the best attainable judgements can be made.

FOUR

Professional Power

One of the main arguments deployed against replacing the NHS by market provision of health care is that the latter would be dominated by a professional monopoly. Professor Maynard, for instance, contends that it is 'naive and unhelpful' to assert that the market is more efficient than the NHS:

'The power of the monopoly interests and the income losses these interests would suffer if competition existed, make it likely that any market for health care will be dominated by monopolies'.[1]

According to Professor Culyer:

'It seems that a strongly organised professional monopoly that controls entry to the profession, terms of service, permitted forms of advertising, disciplinary procedure, etc., is a *universal* characteristic of all developed countries (wherever they lie on the liberal-collective spectrum)'.[2]

Culyer argues that, because of the tendency of the health-care market to monopoly, there is 'at least a *prima facie* case for introducing a countervailing bargaining power, in the form of the state, in the determination of wages and salaries'.[3] Nicholas Bosanquet's view is similar: the NHS has 'above all . . . been a countervailing force to the medical monopoly'. Moreover, he contends that 'Originally, the most important part of this role was in reducing monopoly power over price'.[4] Bosanquet also believes that the 'NHS setting' offers a better chance of developing independent tests of clinical effectiveness run by third parties. He thinks the necessity for such tests is an especially strong reason for the countervailing power of the NHS.[5]

NHS's 'countervailing power' a myth

This analysis of the NHS as a countervailing power is defective because it neglects two truths. First, professional power in both

---

[1] Maynard [1982], p. 508.

[2] Culyer [1982], p. 37 (emphasis in the original).

[3] *Ibid.*   [4] Bosanquet [1984], p. 49.   [5] *Ibid.*, p. 50.

public and private sectors rests largely upon legal privileges unwisely granted by the state. The restrictive practices of the medical
profession, even when they are not *enforced* by government
agencies, are immune from the general law against restrictive
practices. Secondly, the NHS is itself a very important source of
professional monopoly power.

As my study of the medical market in Britain from the 1830s to
1948 shows, the medical profession constantly sought to restrict
competition. Only the countervailing power of the organised
consumer prevented it. It was only when the medical profession
gained access to the powers of the state that it began to be
successful in its monopolistic aims.[1] Thus, fears that replacing the
NHS by private health-care provision would lead to dominance
by medical monopolists are valid. *They are only valid, however,
because the state has misguidedly enhanced the power of the
organised profession.*

Members of the York school are in no sense apologists for the
medical profession. Professor Maynard, in particular, has pulled
no punches in his discussions of professional regulation. The way
in which the medical profession regulates itself by licensing is, he
says, of 'dubious value'. The 'forces of self-interest permit the
profession to pursue pecuniary and non-pecuniary ends that may
not be in the interests of society'. The result is 'inefficiency', 'inequality' and the continuance of 'unethical practices'.[2] Strangely,
however, Professor Maynard concludes that the solution to these
abuses is the manipulation of 'the institutional arrangements of
health-care systems' to provide 'adequate pecuniary and non-
pecuniary incentives to medical decision-makers'.[3] I have argued
that Professor Maynard has over-estimated the value of re-
arranging incentives within health-care systems like the NHS. A
more radical and direct assault on professional restrictive practices
is required; reform of the NHS will fail without it. Likewise, it
means that the NHS cannot be replaced by superior libertarian
arrangements unless the problem of state reinforcement of professional power is tackled. I now consider professional restrictive
practices under two main headings: entry restrictions and anti-
competitive practices.

(i) Entry Restrictions

Three main types of entry restriction will be discussed: voluntary

---

[1] Green [1984 and forthcoming].

[2] Maynard [1980], pp. 154-55.   [3] *Ibid.*, p. 156.

certification, state certification, and legal reservation of specified tasks to the already certified.

(a) Voluntary Certification

All professions have sought to mark themselves out from their competitors. Usually this has involved the issuing of certificates to persons who have undergone a prescribed course of training laid down by incumbents. This process may be an aid to the consumer. While it will not guarantee that every certified practitioner is competent, it will indicate to the consumer that the holder of the certificate has undergone a specified educational experience.

Training requirements can also be abused. The longer the training period, the less easy it is for newcomers to begin practising. There is consequently a temptation to increase the length of the training period solely to discourage new entrants and thus reduce competition. Since in this respect there is an unavoidable clash between the interests of the (existing) profession and those of customers, it is unlikely that the judgement about how long the training period should be could ever be safely left exclusively to the body of existing practitioners.

The length of a prescribed course of training may be determined by the corpus of knowledge it is desirable for practitioners to acquire before embarking on their careers. Or it may reflect a desire to keep out newcomers. Initially, training requirements may reflect only (or mainly) the desirability of acquiring knowledge. Imperceptibly, however, they may be transformed so as to serve chiefly to deter new entrants. The body of knowledge is likely to be continuously changing, and thus may genuinely require the length of a training course to be increased. Abuse is all the more easy because the line is so difficult to draw. Experience has shown that the temptation to abuse such power has always been too strong for professionals. This danger becomes all the more serious if the regulatory body has been delegated powers of compulsion by the state.

(b) The State and Certification

One strategy adopted by professions from an early date has been to seek government approval for their certificates. This state 'seal of approval' has proved most valuable in attracting business away from non-certified practitioners. State approval of training courses carries two main risks: that of turning the consumer's attention away from the individual characteristics of practitioners, and that of ossifying medical practice in favour of established disciplines.

The first drawback of state certification is that it encourages citizens to make their choice of practitioner according to a potentially misleading criterion. Instead of selecting a doctor for his individual qualities and reputation, the citizen is encouraged to select a *qualified* medical man instead of an *un*qualified one. This diverts the consumer's gaze from direct personal to artificial institutional considerations. Moreover, to the extent that the shift of emphasis to 'qualifications' rather than 'qualities' encourages citizens to believe that 'qualified' medical practitioners are all much the same, state interference in certification tends to mislead rather than aid choice.

Preventing fraud without enhancing professional power

There is a legitimate role for government in preventing fraud. Certificates of qualification are plainly of no value to the consumer if they give the impression of competence where it does not exist. To eliminate dubious or fraudulent qualifications is a proper aid to the freedom of the individual. Because of the potentially lethal cost to the consumer of falling into the hands of an incompetent doctor, there is a proper role for government in ensuring that certificates of qualification mean what they say.

The first modern attempt to regulate the medical profession was the 1858 Medical Act, which was based on principles still embodied in today's legislation. Before it was enacted, more than 20 bodies issued medical qualifications and, as T. H. Huxley, the noted liberal thinker and former physician, showed, standards of certification varied widely:

'... there were twenty-one licensing bodies ... They were partly universities, partly medical guilds and corporations, partly the Archbishop of Canterbury. There was no central authority, there was nothing to prevent any one of these licensing authorities from granting a licence to anyone upon any conditions it thought fit. The examination might be a sham, the curriculum might be a sham, the certificate might be bought and sold like anything in a shop; or, on the other hand, the examination might be fairly good and the diploma correspondingly valuable; but there was not the smallest guarantee, except the personal character of the people who composed the administration of each of these licensing bodies, as to what might happen. It was possible for a young man to come to London and to spend two years and six months of the time of his compulsory three years "walking the hospitals" in idleness or worse; he could then, by putting himself in the hands of a judicious "grinder" for the remaining six months, pass triumphantly through the ordeal of one hour's *viva voce* examination, which was all that was absolutely necessary, to enable him to be turned loose upon the public, like Death on the pale horse, "conquering and to conquer", with the full sanction of the law, as a "qualified practitioner".'[1]

---

[1] T. H. Huxley [1884], pp. 230-1, quoted in J. L. Berlant [1975], pp. 158-9.

The method chosen in the 1858 Act was not to abolish the licensing bodies, nor to replace them by a state examining body, but to superimpose over them a General Medical Council (GMC) charged with reviewing each qualification and pronouncing it sound or unsound. This approach satisfied liberal opinion at the time. It did not seem to impose *one* standard of certification, or *one* entry qualification. It permitted several licensing bodies to co-exist in competition, whilst providing a mechanism which enabled misleading qualifications to be eliminated. There is no automatic libertarian objection to this arrangement. And, in the particular situation, it probably served to strengthen the hand of the consumer by improving the reliability of the information at his disposal. But it was not long before the GMC began to impose a single course of training and a single entry requirement, prescribed and enforced by professional incumbents. There had long been pressure for a unified course of training, but the turning point came in the 1880s. In 1884 the Royal College of Physicians and the Royal College of Surgeons instituted joint examinations; and the 1886 Medical Act required doctors to be qualified in both medicine and surgery, thus ending one of the traditional sources of rivalry (and competition).

Today the GMC comprises 95 members. Eleven are nominated by the Privy Council, two of whom must be doctors and nine lay persons. All other members of the GMC are doctors. Fifty members, an overall majority, are elected by the general body of medical practitioners in the UK, whilst the remainder (also doctors) are appointed by the university medical schools or the royal colleges. Because of the difficulty faced by individual doctors in establishing a national reputation, the elections are dominated by the nominees of the British Medical Association—the doctors' 'trade union'.

All state regulation presents the same problem. Once a body has been given powers of regulation for ostensibly valid reasons—in this instance, to eliminate fraud—it is very difficult to ensure that it continues to use those powers in a disinterested manner. The central difficulty is how to maintain the impartiality of a regulatory body like the GMC. It is vital that a state review of qualifications as an aid to consumers is carried out by impartial judges, charged with acting in the public interest and not in the narrow interest of the producer.

This problem is the same for the enforcement of law generally. In the main, the judges have administered the law impartially, and valuable lessons can be learnt from the courts. However, despite the existence of a legal basis on which judges could have prevented the powers of the GMC from being abused, they have failed to use it. The power of the GMC to strike doctors from the medical register for crime or professional misconduct was tempered by Section 52 of the 1858 Act which laid down that:

'Provided always that nothing herein contained shall extend to authorise Her Majesty to create any new restriction in the practice of medicine or surgery, or to grant to any of the said corporations any powers or privileges contrary to the common law of the land'.

The courts have, however, failed to intervene, taking the view that professional misconduct was a matter exclusively for the profession (below, p. 49). Perhaps this has been so because judges are members of a like-minded profession.

The suppression of medical sub-disciplines

The second difficulty with state certification is that it has been usual to distinguish between the qualified and the unqualified, thus implying that those without the state-approved certificate were not qualified in any respect. In practice, many practitioners of healing not included in the Medical Register established under the 1858 Medical Act were highly qualified, but they were not qualified in the officially approved manner. Many unregistered practitioners continued to enjoy public confidence until the 1911 National Insurance Act excluded them from the panel system. A government survey of 1910 suggested that many citizens turned to 'unqualified' medical practitioners. In 82 out of 217 towns studied, unqualified medical practice was either increasing or taking place on a large scale; and it existed to some extent in a further 75 towns. It included chemists who prescribed over the counter, herbalists, bonesetters, Christian Scientists, faith healers, abortionists, and VD specialists. In mining areas such as Northumberland, Durham and Wales, bonesetters enjoyed equal standing with doctors.[1]

Giving a state stamp of approval to one group of qualified persons and not to others was therefore misleading and dangerous. That some qualifications were recognised whilst others were not was more a reflection of the political power of the successful groups than of the relative value of their services to the public. In practice, it discouraged the development of valuable medical disciplines.

Initially, the tightening up which resulted from the GMC review procedure of 1858 was an improvement and conformed with liberal principles to an important extent. But, gradually, the effect

---

[1] PMSUP [1910], pp. 3-4, 8.

of granting power to the organised profession became harmful. For many years disciplines with much to offer medical practice have been denied the state seal of approval because the machinery is dominated by orthodox medicine. Homeopathy, herbalism, acupuncture, osteopathy and chiropractic, among others, have enjoyed public confidence and survived critical scrutiny over many years. Yet, even though their practitioners often undergo rigorous training, they have been excluded from the 'qualified'. According to the Institute for Complementary Medicine (ICM), training in acupuncture, osteopathy, naturopathy, chiropractic, herbal medicine and homeopathy takes from two to six years, depending on the particular discipline. Part-time as well as full-time courses are available, providing an essential grounding in the medical sciences followed by supervised clinical work.[1]

A measure of the public esteem in which alternative medicine is held is that large numbers of citizens pay private fees to consult alternative specialists whose advice is generally unavailable through the NHS. That the patient is, in effect, paying twice for his health care has not prevented a considerable growth in alternative medicine.

A survey carried out in December 1983 by the ICM estimated that there were around 2,000 registered practitioners in the six main alternative therapies—osteopathy, chiropractic, herbal medicine, acupuncture, homeopathy, naturopathy—who carried out around 4·6 million consultations a year. Consultations were claimed to be on the increase.[2]

The issues surrounding certification cannot be resolved simply. No state regulation of any kind might well produce harmful results for patients, the chief danger being fraudulent claims to competence. Government should not enforce a uniform pattern of training, for this would be too open to abuse by producers at a high cost to patients. But it might seek to check fraud in the form of unwarranted claims to the possession of skill or knowledge. This is a wider interpretation of fraud than tends to be ordinarily applied by the courts, but it is legitimate. The underlying principle is that no doctor should mislead a patient into accepting treatment from him unless he has satisfactorily equipped himself to offer his services. This would include undergoing suitable training and making conscientious efforts to keep up to date with new developments.

Once a case for government regulation has been conceded, however, the classical liberal dilemma arises: the state machine,

---

[1] ICM [1984], p. 8.   [2] *Ibid.*, p. 18.

however justified the initial granting of its protective powers, can all too easily turn from protection to depredation. It is vital to recognise that this danger is inherent in all schemes for state regulation. There are two main considerations. First, regulation should never be undertaken lightly: a proper calculation of the risks and benefits of non-regulation should be made and contrasted with the costs and benefits of various types of regulation. Secondly, any scheme of regulation should be designed, not only to prohibit or discourage the particular mischief which initially justified it, but also to prohibit or discourage abuse of the powers granted to the regulatory agency.

In the case of medical certification, the risks and benefits of the existing scheme of regulation have never been fully appraised. The Merrison Committee's Report of 1975, though intended to inquire into the regulation of the medical profession, failed to investigate any of the fundamental issues. Indeed, if anything, it helped to obscure the true character of the current regulatory scheme. The Report comments that an 'instructive' way of looking at regulation

> 'is to see it as a contract between public and profession, by which the public go to the profession for medical treatment because the profession has made sure it will provide satisfactory treatment'.[1]

But, as Professor Klein has observed, 'it is doubtful whether [the GMC] can guarantee "satisfactory treatment" '.[2] The Merrison Committee, however, insisted on referring to the medical register as a register of the competent; and, worse still, it asserted that the body regulating the profession *must* be independent'.[3] The medical register is manifestly *not* a register of the competent; and the GMC is manifestly *not* independent, but rather dominated by the producer.

The risks and benefits of non-regulation

What do we know about the risks and benefits of non-regulation? Before 1858 there were several voluntary certification agencies whose standards varied. Initially, the 1858 Act probably helped to raise standards in the less proficient agencies. Gradually, however, the GMC was transformed from a protective into a predatory agency, advancing professional interests at the expense of patients.

---

[1] Merrison [1975], p. 3.

[2] Klein [1982], p. 107.

[3] Merrison, *op. cit.*, p. 5 (emphasis added).

Moreover, the present arrangements are far from guaranteeing that every registered practitioner is competent, as studies carried out by the Royal College of General Practitioners have repeatedly shown. A study published in October 1984, for instance, revealed that a disturbingly high proportion of GPs were unaware of all the common symptoms of some conditions regularly encountered in general practice. A random sample of GPs was asked a series of questions, one of which was: 'What are the symptoms of acute otitis media?' Examiners at medical finals would expect a correct answer to include pain, discharge and deafness. Yet only about a half of the GP respondents mentioned all three symptoms. In general, the investigators found that 'many respondents failed to mention answers that were important'; some gave 'unusual answers, and some gave answers that were clearly wrong'.[1]

A recent study of hospital doctors found still more disturbing results. A survey of junior hospital doctors practising at the Addenbrooke's Hospital in Cambridge revealed that only 8 per cent were able to manage a cardiopulmonary resuscitation adequately. The author of the report, himself a doctor, concluded that standards were 'scandalously low'. Many hospital patients have undoubtedly died from heart attacks as a result of the 'confused and disorganised charades' conducted during efforts to save them.[2]

Compared with the situation in the non-state sector before the foundation of the NHS in 1948, and especially in the medical market-place before the panel system was introduced in 1913, the lack of competition between doctors which has been a feature of both state schemes may have produced a deterioration in medical competence. Before 1911, the selection of a practitioner was left to consumers to a far greater extent. As we have seen, there were a large number of 'unqualified' practitioners who commanded public confidence. What was the balance of good and harm in this situation? No doubt some individuals made bad choices. But set against this risk was the effect of competition on the conduct of doctors and on prices. Medical fees were very much lower before the panel system was introduced. And the institutions which emerged to provide medical care for the mass of the people helped to encourage good medical practice. The schemes of 1913 and 1948 had relatively little effect on the initial training of doctors, but pressures tending to encourage continued competence *after* initial training were much modified. Doctors are more likely to keep up to date and to continue improving their

---

[1] H. W. K. Acheson and M. H. Henley [1984], p. 23.
[2] *The Times*, 15 January 1985.

knowledge and skills if benefits accrue to them for doing so and if undesirable consequences befall the incompetent. As my study of the pre-NHS medical market-place shows, the doctor with a reputation for incompetence or inattention quickly found himself with few patients. And the doctor who, without being incompetent, nonetheless fell short of the standards desired by consumers faced an effective disciplinary procedure. There are parallels today. In Denmark there is no regulation requiring that only doctors or opticians may carry out sight-testing; anyone may do it. And because there is competition, no detectable harmful results have emerged. The syndicalism of the NHS makes the emergence of such incentives in the state sector highly unlikely.

What price to avoid incompetence?

What price is it worth paying to reduce the chances of patients falling into the hands of incompetent doctors? Most people would accept the necessity for some regulation (with its inevitable loss of liberty) to deter incompetents or charlatans. But present arrangements go far beyond this step; and they do *not*, moreover, eliminate low-calibre doctors. In the end, there is no substitute for the diligence of the consumer. Laws should reinforce the diligent consumer, not seek to replace him.

The problem for the would-be state regulator is to find a method of pronouncing impartially on the wide variety of qualifications available without at the same time ossifying conditions and thus favouring current insiders at the expense of outsiders. This is unlikely to be accomplished if regulation is carried out by representatives of established disciplines.

Powers of a reformed GMC

A reformed regulatory agency ought not, therefore, to be dominated by representatives of orthodox medicine. While its powers compared with the present GMC should be significantly curtailed, it could be charged with carrying out impartial reviews of the variety of qualifications on offer to prospective practitioners of healing. Its members should be required to act in a strictly non-sectional manner, and to issue reports which fearlessly state facts and make recommendations to citizens. Individuals would be free to place their trust in the new agency's pronouncements or to reject them as they saw fit.

A new agency could continue to be called the General Medical Council, but a name like the Medical Certification Association

(MCA) would probably be better. There could be no guarantee, of course, that such a new agency would not fall into the hands of self-interested producer groups. For this reason it should enjoy no powers of coercion or exclusion. Unlike the GMC, it should have no authority to close down training courses. However, the publication of an unfavourable report by the MCA could be expected to have a strong effect on the organisers of any course of training. To ensure easier access for emerging disciplines, the new agency should be specifically charged with investigating them without prejudice.

One question remains. Why should faith be placed in any state regulatory agency, even with the safeguards outlined? Apart from the risk of the agency falling into the self-interested hands of producers,[1] there is well-documented evidence from America demonstrating that a politicised regulatory process has an inherent tendency to over-regulation.[2] This happens because the potential political *gains* from *over*-regulation and the political *costs* of *under*-regulation are both very high. There is thus a natural tendency towards excessive interference. The unnecessarily time-consuming regulation of the US pharmaceutical industry, for instance, has meant that some new medicines have failed to reach ill Americans as quickly as citizens of less-regulated countries. Americans have undoubtedly died as a result.

Some analysts maintain that, even though the market is imperfect, its imperfections are a lot less costly than the imperfections of state regulation.[3] And the market clearly does regulate, not only through voluntary systems of formal regulation within an industry but by eliminating unsatisfactory suppliers. The disadvantage is that the market acts after the event. Consumers exposed directly or indirectly to bad-quality products withdraw their support and unsuccessful suppliers must improve their performance or go out of business. But by then the damage has been done. Medicine presents a special problem in that the citizen exposed to a low-calibre doctor may die or suffer permanent disability as a result. For this reason, consumers have long sought means by which incompetent suppliers could be eliminated before they did any harm.

Eliminating incompetents

Plainly, this end can never be perfectly accomplished; and cer-

---

[1] For a short but masterly analysis, George J. Stigler, *The Pleasures and Pains of Modern Capitalism*, 13th Wincott Memorial Lecture, Occasional Paper 64, IEA, 1982.

[2] M. and R. Friedman [1980].   [3] *Ibid.*

tainly it has been a grave mistake to believe that professional self-regulation was the best way of preventing misfortune before it happened. In view of the unsatisfactory track-record of 'pre-emptive' methods of regulation, is it advisable to abandon all pre-emptive regulation? Or can new techniques be devised which do not impose the same costs? I will argue that the potentially very high costs to patients of low-calibre medical practitioners demand an attempt to devise new pre-emptive regulatory methods. Two principles should be applied. First, the new regulatory agency should not undermine the market's own methods of eliminating incompetents. And, secondly, regulators should seek to strengthen the hand of the diligent consumer by placing additional information about practitioners at his or her disposal.

How will the members of a new regulatory agency be chosen? And how will they be constrained to perform their duties im-partially? There is a parallel here with the problem faced by clubs or associations. Whilst different factions will control the manage-ment committee over a period of time, members do not usually wish the accumulated funds of the club to be wholly at the disposal of the controlling faction of the day. To prevent this result and to ensure the general propriety of all financial dealings, trustees are appointed to control the funds. Trustees have a well-defined legal role: they must not, for example, profit from their trust, they must not as a general rule delegate their duties, and they must produce accounts for inspection. If they contravene the trust, an action for damages may lie against them and in some circumstances they may be criminally liable.

The duties of a new regulatory agency could be given the same legal standing as the objects of a trust, and the members of the regulatory body could be placed under the same constraints as trustees. In particular, the requirement that no member should profit from the performance of his duties should rule out the participation of any practising doctor.

The principal current abuses could thus be avoided. Fraudulent claims to proficiency could be policed without the high risk of ossifying medicine in favour of established or orthodox interests.

(c) Legal Reservation of Specified Tasks

Professor Milton Friedman has identified three main regulatory devices: registration, or keeping a list of all doctors in practice; certification, or keeping a list of all who have obtained a specified (voluntary) qualification; and licensure, or requiring every person who wishes to pursue an occupation to obtain a licence from the state. The method chosen in 1858 was certification. As we have seen, certification was harmful because it seemed to give doctors on the medical register a kind of government stamp of approval when, in reality, inclusion on the register had only a tenuous connection with competence. But persons not on the medical register were still allowed to practise healing, and did so in large numbers.

Unfortunately, the 1858 Act also began the process of reserving certain tasks for government-certified practitioners. It required medical officers serving benefit societies and poor law medical officers to be on the medical register. The reservation of tasks was extended in 1911: only doctors on the medical register were allowed to serve insured members of the public under the government national insurance scheme. In 1917, the unqualified were forbidden to attend people suffering from venereal disease. And in 1920, the Dangerous Drugs Act laid down restrictions which meant that only doctors on the medical register could obtain and hold specified drugs essential to the effective practice of medicine. The 1939 Cancer Act forbade anyone except registered medical practitioners from treating cancer patients, and the 1941 Pharmacy and Medicines Act banned unregistered practitioners from treating a long list of diseases which included diabetes, epilepsy and tuberculosis. When the NHS was founded in 1948, only practitioners on the medical register were permitted to serve in it, thus reducing still further the scope for uncertified practitioners.

The reservation of positions in the state medical service for doctors on rhe medical register was vitally important to the medical profession. The main turning point was 1911. Before then, large numbers of non-orthodox medical practitioners offered their services successfully. After national insurance panel practice was reserved for orthodox medicine, it became very much more difficult for other disciplines to survive.

Other tasks continue to be reserved for registered medical practitioners today. The most important are:

1. Under the 1983 Medical Act (section 47), only registered medical practitioners may serve in the naval, military, or air service, in any hospital not supported wholly by voluntary contributions, and in any prison, public institution, or friendly society.

2. Under the 1977 National Health Service Act (s.31 (1) (a)), only persons of 'suitable experience' may provide general medical services for the NHS. The Minister can issue regulations about

what constitutes suitable experience but, effectively, only registered practitioners (and those similarly qualified overseas) are included.

3. Registered medical practitioners are the only persons entitled to prescribe, hold or supply a large list of medicines vital to modern medical care. Controlled drugs under the 1971 Misuse of Drugs Act may be prescribed only by doctors (and, in some cases, by dentists and veterinary surgeons). The supply and possession of drugs is also restricted to doctors and other specified persons. Under the Medicines Act of 1968, the Minister lays down which medicines shall be on the general sales list and which shall not. Under that Act (s.55), doctors—together with registered pharmacists, dentists, hospitals, registered nurses (in some instances) and vets (again, in some instances)—may sell or supply medicines not on the general sales list. (Herbalists enjoy limited exemption under s.56.) The Minister can lay down which medicines are available only on prescription from doctors—and, in some cases, from dentists and vets (s.58).

4. Only a registered medical practitioner may issue a certificate of cause of death. (Births and Deaths Registration Act, 1953, s.22(2), s.41; Medical Act 1983, s.48.)

5. Dentistry is reserved for dentists and doctors under the Dentists Act of 1984 (s.38).

6. Sight-testing is reserved for opticians and doctors under the 1958 Opticians Act (s.20).

Prevention of abuse

How can abuse by registered medical practitioners of these legal requirements be prevented? The monopoly of prescribing presents a particular problem. There are two main reasons for making drugs available only on prescription: (i) to inhibit criminal misuse of medicines, and (ii) to prevent patients from taking medicines without first obtaining advice. It is the second that is most susceptible to abuse. Let us concede that patients ought to seek the fullest information before taking medicines since they may be unaware of possible side-effects or of the possible consequences of mixing one drug with another or with certain kinds of food and drink. An individual's view about regulating access to medicines for the self-protection of the patient depends upon his values. A libertarian would hold that, even though a patient would be foolish to take medicines without first seeking advice, this is no reason for the state to ban access to drugs. The state may caution the patient, but banning access for the patient's self-protection is objectionable.

One way of cautioning citizens without legally banning access to drugs would be to require them to sign a statement at the chemist's shop before they could receive items on a given list. The statement would verify that the patient had taken advice or obtained information and fully understood the likely effects of the drug he was buying and its possible side-effects.

Restricting access to medicines

Medicine without knowledge can do a patient more harm than good. It is therefore irresponsible to supply a medicine without also supplying the vital information about how best to use it. Government can properly require anyone supplying drugs to accompany them with the requisite information. But this can be achieved without giving a monopoly to incumbent suppliers.

An alternative procedure would be for a reformed GMC to keep separate lists of drugs which could be prescribed by each approved discipline: one for orthodox medicine, one for herbalists, one for osteopaths, acupuncturists, and so on. This would be an extension of the present arrangement under which the Minister keeps separate lists for doctors, dentists, and veterinary surgeons. The new regulatory agency should meet two requirements. First, it should be charged with keeping lists as short as possible: only medicines which present an exceptionally high risk to patients should be available solely on prescription, and as few medicines as possible should be obtainable only through pharmacies. Secondly, when the risks of taking a particular medicine are felt to justify compelling citizens to go to a limited group of previously designated suppliers (such as doctors or pharmacists), the new agency should ensure that no potential suppliers who are fit to prescribe or supply medicines are excluded. I return to this second requirement below (p. 48).

Many people will doubtless feel uneasy about adopting such a course because they are aware there are very many drugs and they know very little about the side-effects and risks associated with them. From the knowledge that each of us is ignorant about *most* medicines, it is tacitly inferred that we are ignorant about *every* medicine. Yet, if they are consuming medicine at all, most people are taking only one or two preparations at any moment. And in most instances it is a very simple matter to acquire the essential information about those medicines. Acquiring knowledge is largely a matter of incentives. Few of us have the time or inclination to find out about the risks associated with drugs we are unlikely ever to take. But we have a very consideranle incentive to master the rules or body of facts associated with a medicine we are advised to take. This is what J. S. Mill meant when he wrote:

'with respect to his own feelings and circumstances, the most ordinary man or woman has means of knowledge immeasurably surpassing those that can be possessed by anyone else'.[1]

And it is what Edmund Burke had in mind when he remarked:

'in my course I have known, and, according to my measure, have co-operated with great men; and I have never yet seen any plan which has not been mended by the observations of those who were much inferior in their understanding to the person who took the lead in the business'.[2]

To suggest that fewer medicines should be obtainable only on prescription is not to suppose that every patient knows as much as every doctor about the whole array of alternative drugs. It supposes only that most people can and do rapidly absorb the essential facts about the few medicines which may benefit them or which they are already taking. Indeed, the patient has a stronger incentive than the doctor to exercise caution, for it is the patient who will suffer any side-effects. Moreover, there is a tendency to over-estimate the reliability of the knowledge possessed by doctors.

There have been a number of surveys on the sources of doctors' information about drugs. A 1976 survey of 453 medical prac-titioners found that the *Monthly Index of Medical Specialities* (*MIMS*) was the most popular source of information used during consultations: 77 per cent of respondents referred to it to select an appropriate drug for treatment and 96 per cent to check on dosage and/or strength. Three out of four doctors also used it to check on adverse effects and contra-indications (circumstances in which a drug should not be prescribed). *MIMS* is, however, an abbreviated guide which, at the time of the survey, did not list adverse effects and provided only incomplete information about contra-indications.[3]

A survey of 398 doctors carried out for the Office of Health Economics in 1975 asked them to state which sources they considered most important to gain information about both new and established medicines. For new medicines, pharmaceutical company representatives were mentioned by 33 per cent of

---

[1] Mill [1861], p. 133.

[2] Burke [1907], vol. 4, p. 187.

[3] G. Eaton and P. Parish [1976], pp. 60-61.

respondents—more frequently than any other source. Next came articles in medical journals, mentioned by 17 per cent. For established medicines, *MIMS* was mentioned most frequently—by 23 per cent of respondents. Second were articles in medical journals, with 19 per cent.[1]

Some critics favour the control of access to drugs through prescriptions because they believe that many of their fellow citizens would otherwise start swallowing tablets and swigging medicines as if they were confectionery. But I suspect that quite the reverse would happen. If more of us made the (not very considerable) effort to become better informed about the risks connected with particular medicines, and were less inclined to surrender our judgement to doctors, we would swallow far less medicine.

It is also claimed that some citizens are easily confused and find it difficult to cope with the burden of choice—which is certainly true of some people. But is it in the interests of people who prefer to rely wholly on the advice of others that they should be compelled to rely only on the advice of a monopolistic medical profession? It is arguable that their interests would be better served if advice was available to them from a variety of sources—including, crucially, people not actively involved on the supply side—for a range of sources of advice is infinitely preferable to one source. Present arrangements take insufficient account of the propensity of the medical profession for self-interested conduct.

Should paternalistic protection be the rule?

Those who favour paternalistic protection of the consumer frequently identify the elderly as a group which will become confused and whose health will suffer if the burden of choice falls more heavily on them. The elderly are also said to be particularly 'bad' at taking their medicines correctly. No doubt some elderly patients who are prescribed multiple drugs do get confused and require sympathetic help. But many who fail to take their medicines as directed do so not because they are confused but because they mistrust either their doctor or the medicines. This is not necessarily unwise, and many elderly persons may owe their longevity to it. The difficulty facing anyone who does not trust either his doctor or the drugs he prescribes is that open expression of such a sentiment may produce resentment; it is much wiser to portray oneself as confused and thus to provoke professional pity rather

---

[1] OHE [1977], pp. 17-18.

than anger. Estimates vary of the proportion of prescriptions either never collected from the chemists or not consumed as directed, but the likely figure is between one-third and one-half. This phenomenon frequently arises because patients mistrust the medicines prescribed. Doctors often contend that patients put them under pressure to prescribe; patients are said to feel 'cheated' if they leave a surgery without a prescription. No doubt this is true of some patients. But doctors also use the handing over of a prescription as a device to signify the end of the consultation and to speed the patient on his way. Furthermore, it is not uncommon for patients to accept a prescription merely to humour the doctor, only to refrain from having it dispensed or from taking it if it is made up.

The second duty of the new regulatory agency would be to ensure that prescribing rights were divided among the various disciplines according to an impartial view of the knowledge at the disposal of each. Many drugs, therefore, would appear on the lists of several disciplines. No single discipline should be allowed to dominate the allocation with the risk that prescribing rights for vital medicines could be denied to competitors so as to diminish the value of such competition to patients. As a safeguard against abuse, the lists should be registered as restrictive trade practices and be subject to the jurisdiction of the Restrictive Practices Court.

(ii) Contrivances to Restrict Competition

Contrivances to restrict competition may take three forms: (a) voluntary contrivances; (b) restrictive practices enforced by the state; and (c) restrictive practices not enforced, but *permitted* by the state as a result of its granting immunities from general laws which prohibit agreements in restraint of trade.

Voluntary certification of members of a profession has usually been taken to require the enforcement of a code of conduct as well as of entry qualifications. This power can be abused. A rule of conduct, which may be justified in some circumstances in order to protect consumers, can easily (and perhaps imperceptibly) be transformed into a restrictive practice intended to reduce or eliminate competition.

At least in part, professional codes of conduct have invariably acted as codes of restrictive practices designed to restrain competition. As with entry restrictions, the damage that may result is increased if the profession has at its disposal the coercive power of the state.

The 1858 Act gave the GMC the power to regulate the conduct of doctors on the medical register (in addition to the power to review training courses). Doctors could be struck from the medical register if convicted of a criminal offence or if they were found guilty of 'infamous conduct in a professional respect'. Thus the GMC could deny a doctor the opportunity of earning his livelihood if, for example, he refused to co-operate with professional restrictive practices designed to inhibit competition and raise prices. From 1901 it put this power to effective use.

It is a great tribute to the integrity of the majority of doctors on the GMC that they resisted many years of pressure from the wider medical profession to use the powers of the GMC to advance the pecuniary interests of doctors. It was not until the decisions of 1901 and 1902 to ban canvassing and advertising that the profession succeeded in seriously abusing the powers of the GMC.[1] The bans on canvassing and advertising, still in force today, have the effect of limiting the information at the disposal of consumers, thereby making it difficult to establish the vital differences between individual practitioners who naturally vary considerably in skill, knowledge and attentiveness.

Professional misconduct

The role and powers of the GMC have changed little over the years. Under the Medical Act of 1983 (s.36(1)), its disciplinary committee can erase or suspend an entry in the medical register if a doctor is found guilty of a criminal offence or is judged to have been guilty of 'serious professional misconduct'.[2]

Professional misconduct was defined in 1894 by Lord Justice Lopes:

> 'If a medical man in the pursuit of his profession has done something with regard to it which will be reasonably regarded as disgraceful or dishonourable by his professional brethren of good repute and competency, then it is open to the General Medical Council, if that be shown, to say that he has been guilty of infamous conduct in a professional respect'.[3]

A judgement delivered by Lord Justice Scrutton in 1930 passed the buck even more succinctly:

> 'Infamous conduct in a professional respect means no more than serious misconduct judged according to the rules, written or unwritten, governing the profession'.[4]

---

[1] Green [forthcoming].

[2] The offence was called 'infamous conduct in a professional respect' until the 1969 Medical Act (s.13(1)).

[3] GMC [1983], pp. 2-3.

[4] *Ibid.*

Professional misconduct has, therefore, been interpreted as exclusively a matter for the profession. Consequently, the GMC has done little to protect consumers. In addition, doctors have been singularly unwilling to testify against each other in disciplinary cases—a problem which has not diminished with time. The Merrison Committe felt there was evidence that *unthinking* mutual loyalty may be on the increase'.[1]

The Committee also found that:

'It was not the duty or practice of any professional body to collect evidence of misconduct or to prosecute proceedings. The Medical Defence Societies occasionally assumed the role, but only in relation to advertising or canvassing by doctors not members of the society and where it was felt the action complained of was prejudicial to the interests of their own members'.[2]

It is not my argument that advertising requires no regulation whatsoever; some control is necessary to protect the consumer. There can be no objection to doctors publicising their prices to compete with other doctors. And there can be no objection to doctors announcing their special skills or experience. But the consumer is entitled to the protection of the law against fraudulent claims to expertise. To date, this protection has been offered by means of professional self-regulation. And the outcome has been the banning of *all* advertising deliberately to make it difficult for consumers to differentiate between doctors in any significant respects. More fitting would have been regulation by means of the general law, for example, a civil law prohibiting fraudulent or unsupportable claims to competence which provided for civil remedies. Any doctor who advertised his services as, say, 'Only £5 per Consultation; Cure Guaranteed' could thus be sued not for advertising his fee but for claiming that a cure was guaranteed when no such claim could reasonably be made.

The British Medical Association (BMA)—the doctors' trade union—has also sought to enforce other restrictive agreements (though it has not had the help of the GMC in every respect). Throughout its history it has attempted to enforce uniform fees, although with little success until the state medical service came along in 1911. In the market, high fees were very difficult to obtain; governments, able to turn to the ever-pliant taxpayer, have been much easier to coerce. Although doctors' pay is largely negotiated with government today, the BMA still tries to impose uniform fees on the small private sector (there are, for instance, fees for medical examinations which are not covered by the NHS).

The BMA has also sought to ban certain types of practice. At

---

[1] Merrison [1975], p. 82.   [2] *Ibid.*, p. 86.

one stage it particularly opposed salaried service under the control of lay committees, and sought the support of the GMC. The BMA was especially hostile to the medical institutes run by friendly societies and the medical aid societies run by Welsh miners.[1]

Immunity from general law

The medical profession, in common with other professions, has not only sought special laws to enhance its power; it has also sought immunity from general laws which impeded its efforts to advance its interests. It has particularly sought immunity from laws governing restrictive practices.

Before there were statutes governing monopolies and restrictive practices, the courts intervened by applying a general prohibition on 'restraints of trade'. This had only a patchy effect on the medical profession. In 1948 came the first statute, the Monopolies & Restrictive Practices (Inquiries Control) Act, which established the Monopolies Commission. It was followed in 1956 by the Restrictive Trade Practices Act which established a Court to regulate restrictive practices in the supply of goods. Until 1965, the legislation did not apply to services, and the professions could be touched by neither the Monopolies Commission nor the Restrictive Practices Court. But under the Monopolies & Mergers Act of that year, the powers of the Monopolies Commission were extended to services, and in 1970 the Commission produced a report dealing with restrictive practices in the professions. Although it led to a series of reports on particular professions, the medical profession has survived unscathed.

It was not until the 1973 Fair Trading Act that the Restrictive Practices Court was given jurisdiction over restrictive agreements in services—but the professions were excluded (as they continued to be under the 1976 Restrictive Trade Practices Act (s.13, Schedule 1)). The 1973 Act also excluded the medical profession from consumer protection legislation.[2]

(iii) The NHS as a Source of Professional Power

The NHS enhances the power of the organised medical profession at the expense of the consumer. The delivery of health care in

---

[1] Green [forthcoming]; also the 'Historical Postscript', below, p. 60 *et seq.*

[2] Under section 14, any consumer trade practice which adversely affects the economic interests of consumers can be referred to the Consumer Protection Advisory Committee. The medical profession is among the professions excluded in Schedule 4 of the Act.

kind, financed by compulsory taxation, deprives all but the most wealthy citizens (or those with a generous employer) of the resources to pay for alternative methods of health care. A state monopoly in which consumers are stripped of their purchasing power, forced to pay for whatever they are given, and with negligible competition among suppliers, is potentially more harmful than a private-sector monopoly faced by at least the prospect of competition. Total expenditure on health care is fixed at the whim of government.

The result is prolonged and unnecessary suffering and even premature death for many patients. Two recent scandals have brought this reality vividly to public attention. In a case which is not an isolated incident, doctors denied dialysis to kidney patient Derek Sage and sent him home expecting him to die within days. And at about the same time the Government proposed to restrict the drugs available to NHS patients to a limited list, widely criticised as inadequate to cater for all medical needs. This is not a problem peculiar to the present Government. Ever since 1948, expenditure on health care in Britain has been below what citizens would probably have chosen to spend had they been left in control of their own resources. The imposition of a state medical service has weakened each citizen's control of his or her destiny.

Through the democratic process, governments are supposed to represent the consumers' interests. In reality, governments find themselves forced to make concessions to organised producer groups—trade union, professional and others. In 1911, when the panel system laid the foundations of the NHS, and again in 1946, government needed the co-operation of the medical profession. A high price was demanded by doctors, and successive governments agreed to pay up.[1] Equally as serious, the monopoly position of the NHS, resting as it does on the awesome powers vested by law in the Minister, has made it virtually impossible for the Monopolies Commission to interfere with the power of the medical profession. Professional monopoly power is an integral part of the NHS monopoly; but the NHS, and particularly the Minister responsible for it, are beyond the reach of the Commission.

---

[1] Green [1982], [1984 and forthcoming].

FIVE

Conclusions and Proposals

Conclusions

The recently-advanced view that the NHS offers advantages not so much on the demand but rather on the supply side is defective. Any effort to re-structure the NHS in order to manipulate the environment in which doctors function in the hope of inducing different, and particularly less self-interested, professional conduct is likely to fail. Such measures will not succeed unless professional monopoly is replaced by competition among doctors. But the chief barriers to competition have been erected by the state. Unless those barriers are eliminated first, significant reform of the NHS will be stifled by either open or covert professional resistance.

Those who favour the extension of the private sector in health face a similar dilemma. The expansion of the existing private sector may produce small improvements here and there, but it will not necessarily help to diminish the monopoly power of the profession. A precondition of significant reform of health care in Britain is the elimination of state-imposed barriers to competition.

(i) A Non-Sectional State?

Why has state regulation of the medical profession so often benefited producers at the expense of consumers? The underlying reason is that governments have failed to take sufficient account of the self-seeking character of professionals. Adam Smith's contention that 'People of the same trade seldom meet together, even for merriment and diversion, but the conversation ends in a conspiracy against the public, or in some contrivance to raise prices' is still relevant. He was not in favour of using the law to prevent such meetings. He did, however, argue that, 'though the law cannot hinder people of the same trade from sometimes assembling together, it ought to do nothing to facilitate such assemblies, much less to render them necessary'.[1]

This result is precisely what government policies of regulation

---

[1] Smith [1776], vol. 1, p. 117.

and direct provision of health care have accomplished. The formation of the GMC encouraged professional organisation, and particularly the inclusion on it in 1886 of five members elected by the profession. The Acts of 1911 and 1946 made it even more necessary for doctors to band together in self-defence. Both produced massive lobbying prior to their enactment. The continuing impetus towards both defensive and assertive professional organisation as a consequence of state intervention has been reflected in the steady increase in BMA membership from around 55 per cent in 1911 to over 70 per cent in recent years.[1]

The restoration of a market in medical care would require significant legal reforms to curtail professional monopoly power. Those reforms are summarised below (pp. 55-57). Meanwhile, the problem of establishing and maintaining a non-sectional state calls for some discussion.

We live in the age of the vested interest. Political conflict is dominated by the demands of this or that group for privileges at the general expense. Is it possible that, in the midst of such conflict, agreement to maintain a non-sectional state could be reached? In a pluralistic social order in which wealth and power are unevenly distributed, and in which political struggle is about how to get more of both, is it realistic to suppose that the state could be elevated above the fray?

Historically, inequality has been a central concern in liberal thought. It was one of the principal reasons for opposition to the emergence of a discriminatory or arbitrary state. To put the argument very simply, if there was an unequal distribution of wealth and power, it was all the more important to deny the capacity of the state for coercion to those already well-endowed with political and economic resources. It was believed that, if the state—with its police, its army, and its powers to seize resources—was seen as an instrument available for capture by any section of the population, those who already possessed political and economic power would have a stronger chance of capturing it. Liberals held that it was better to have political conflict about *whether or not* the state should be a tool of this or that vested interest, rather than conflict about *which vested interest* should control the state at any moment. Behind this view lay the belief that there was more chance of securing agreement to deny control of the state to *everyone* than there was of preventing the already powerful from gaining control of the state in a political culture which tolerated self-interested state capture.

---

[1] P. R. Jones [1980].

Today, sectional abuse of state power is taken for granted. But in the to-ing and fro-ing of party political struggle there are few outright winners. If anything, the outcome tends to reflect the prevailing distribution of wealth and power. A society without conflict is virtually inconceivable. But a society in which the parties to conflict *all* agree not to abuse the state machine in particular causes may just be possible.

(ii) A Libertarian Strategy for Regulating the Professions

We have seen that medical (or other) training requirements and entry qualifications can be abused. The length of a training course might reflect the amount of knowledge it was genuinely believed a qualified doctor should possess. Equally, it might reflect a desire to discourage new entrants. Similarly, a professional code of conduct might sometimes offer protection to the consumer, but it might also be transformed into a set of restrictive agreements which act very much against the consumer's interests. The control of medicines raises similar issues.

Some entry restrictions and anti-competitive practices are enforced by professional associations, membership of which is voluntary. And sometimes there is state involvement. Whether the enforcement agency is voluntary or statutory, there are no grounds for it to enjoy legal immunity from general law. To withdraw the current immunity would require the amendment of section 13 of the Restrictive Trade Practices Act of 1976. Schedule 1 of that Act, which lists excluded occupations, should be repealed so that professional restrictive practices would have to be registered. If they remained unchallenged by the Director General of Fair Trading, they would simply continue in being. But if the Director General felt they were against the public interest, he could bring them before the Restrictive Practices Court.

The Court presumes that a restrictive agreement brought before it is against the public interest unless the producer can show otherwise. That is, the burden of proof falls on the producer. If the Court finds an agreement to be against the public interest, it is void in law and the producer is expected to give an undertaking not to devise a similar agreement. The Court can also issue orders prohibiting or modifying agreements.

What would this mean for the restrictive practices of the medical profession? The advertising and canvassing bans would in all likelihood be declared void quite rapidly. Other rules in the professional code of ethics, such as those governing abortions or sexual conduct with patients, would not be brought before the Court.

How would training requirements be dealt with? I have already proposed the establishment of a new impartial body charged with reviewing training courses and pronouncing judgement on them, but without the power to ban them. But an additional safeguard would be advisable—namely, that training requirements should be registered as restrictive agreements which could be referred to the Court if they appeared to be against the public interest. The Court would then have to determine whether the length of a training course was in practice justified by the volume of knowledge to be acquired or whether the training requirements had become a restrictive practice intended to deter potential newcomers.

This approach acknowledges that a good case can often be made, in the interests of consumers, for training requirements and a professional code of ethics. Such recognition has almost certainly led Parliaments to exclude professional regulation from the general law on restrictive practices. But regulations which may be beneficial in some circumstances can come to be abused. And they can become all the more perniciously anti-competitive precisely because they are not wholly without justification.

Policy Proposals

1. The General Medical Council should be abolished and replaced by a body charged with performing impartially a limited set of tasks: (a) to review training requirements and report its findings, though with no power to ban courses; (b) to maintain a register of approved courses, whether general or specialist; (c) to determine which drugs should be available only on prescription and which medical disciplines should prescribe particular drugs.

2. Its members should have the legal status of trustees, liable in law for failure to discharge their duties correctly and forbidden to profit from their activities as trustees.

3. All rulings of the new regulatory agency should be registered as restrictive practices under the 1976 Restrictive Trade Practices Act.

4. All current training requirements should be systematically reviewed to establish whether they are justified by the knowledge it is desirable for practitioners to master.

5. The new regulatory agency should have no role in enforcing a code of conduct; matters such as advertising should be regulated by general law to secure honesty in trading.

6. Legal immunity from restrictive trade practices law under section 13 (Schedule 1) of the 1976 Restrictive Trade Practices Act should be withdrawn.

7. There should be no state medical service in which jobs are reserved for practitioners licensed by the state.

8. The legal reservation of tasks, such as prescribing and issuing death certificates, for specified individuals would be based on the recommendation of the new regulatory agency subject to review by the Restrictive Practices Court.

9. The current list of medicines available only on prescription should be urgently reviewed to establish whether the risk of misuse by criminals or patients is sufficiently serious to justify limiting access, or whether inclusion on the list unnecessarily restricts competition.

10. Legal immunity from consumer protection law under section 14 of the 1973 Fair Trading Act should be withdrawn.

Competition on the Eve of the NHS

ONE

The Family Doctor in the 1930s

Since 1913 national insurance had provided the insured population (largely men in work) with a medical benefit which included the attendance of a GP and the cost of medicines prescribed. By the late-1930s just under half the population was covered. The organised medical profession enjoyed an officially sanctioned monopoly in servicing the insured population, but in the market sector they were not all-powerful. The uninsured population (mainly women and children) secured GP services in a variety of ways. The main types of provision were: the outpatient departments of the voluntary hospitals, the free dispensaries, the provident dispensaries, friendly society lodge practice, friendly society medical institutes, insurance against medical fees, public medical services, private doctors' clubs, and works clubs.

Was there competition in the market sector? And did this have an effect on medical fees? In the 1930s large numbers of people continued to use outpatient departments instead of their GP, even though, under pressure from the BMA (which largely represented GPs), voluntary hospitals were encouraging or even requiring patients to go to their GP first. In 1935 there were 1,013 voluntary hospitals. They admitted 1·2 million inpatients and treated 5·6 million outpatients.[1] Some local authority hospitals performed a similar role.

Free dispensaries, financed by charities, continued to function in many large towns. In the mid-1930s there were over 20 in the London area alone. Provident dispensaries also continued to operate. In the London area there were again almost 20.[2]

A number of private doctors' clubs continued to function after 1913, but it is impossible to estimate how many patients were covered. In the judgement of a BMA survey of 1938-39, it was evident that private clubs were 'gradually dying out'. In the 'great majority' of cases divisional secretaries reported that there were no private clubs. Often they had been absorbed into public medical

---

[1] PEP [1937], p. 231.   [2] *Ibid.*, p. 152.

services.[1] It seems unlikely that more than 100,000 people were covered by private club membership. Many factories and all collieries provided medical attendance. Some were managed by the employer and some by committees representing the workers. Usually, such schemes covered families as well as employees.

The BMA and 'public medical services'

The BMA had been steadily promoting the establishment of 'public medical services'. These were modelled on the provident dispensaries, but differed in that they were run by doctors and not by committees of laymen. The largest was in London, and by 1937 there were 'just below 80' services with 650,000 subscribers throughout the country, covering about 1·2 million people. About 4,000 doctors were involved.[2]

According to the BMA's surveys of contract practice rates carried out in 1935-36 and 1938-39, contract practice to adult members of friendly societies was 'steadily diminishing'. But it was still to be found in many areas.[3]

In 1935 there were 656 registered friendly societies purely for juveniles, with 213,880 members; 87 deposit societies with 2,008,087; 17,213 orders and branches with 2,903,365; 679 dividing societies with 416,831; and 977 unitary societies paying sickness benefit, with 1,140,298 members. Many of these members were not covered for medical benefit. Excluding the deposit societies (which are counted separately), however, there must have been at least 1·2 million persons obtaining medical care and medicines through the societies.[4]

Schemes run on part-payment principles (co-insurance) expanded very rapidly after 1913. In 1936 over 1·3 million members of the National Deposit Friendly Society (NDFS) were covered for payment of a proportion of doctors' bills, as were 57,000 members of the Teachers Provident Society.[5] Until 1948, under the NDFS system members paid 2s 6d for a surgery attendance and 3s 6d for a home visit, including medicine. Payment could be made direct to the doctor or to the member.[6] For male members who had joined between the ages of 16 and 30, 75 per cent of a

---

[1] BMA, General Practice Committee, Documents 1938-39, GP107, pp. 1-6.

[2] *BMJ Supplement*, 10 December 1938, pp. 357-62.

[3] BMA, Medico-Political Committee, Documents 1936-37, MP31, pp. 14-18.

[4] D. G. Green [forthcoming].

[5] PEP, *op. cit.*, p. 154.

[6] NDFS, *Rules*, 1949, rule 91.

doctor's fee was paid by the society. For those who joined between the ages of 5 to 16 or 30 to 40, the society paid two-thirds. The remainder was paid from the member's personal interest-bearing deposit account with the society.[1] According to the BMA, however, a 'considerable number' of doctors accepted the NDFS payment alone in full settlement of the account.[2]

Statistics of medical institutes and societies

Some of the medical institutes and a few Welsh works clubs (the medical aid societies) were 'approved' under the 1911 Act to provide national insurance medical benefit. In Wales in 1924, there were 15 medical aid societies with 39,000 members registered under the 1924 National Health Insurance Act.[3] By 1938 there were still 12 approved institutions covering around 34,000 people, under what had become the National Health Insurance Act of 1936.[4] In 1944 there were 11 approved institutions with 37,000 members.[5]

By 1924, 44 medical institutes in England were affiliated to the Friendly Societies Medical Alliance (FSMA). They had 120,000 insured members, with an additional 41,000 adults receiving attendance plus 60,000 juveniles.[6] In 1929 the FSMA had 142,000 voluntary members, in addition to its 106,000 state members. In 1936, 119,000 insured persons received medical benefit from medical institutes. By 1945 there were 37 approved institutions in England serving 105,000 members.[7]

In 1939 Great Britain had a population of 46·5 million. Of these, about 19 million were covered by national insurance. Outpatient departments of both voluntary and public hospitals must have served about 6 million; the charitable and provident dispensaries perhaps 300,000; the lodges 1·2 million; the medical institutes 150,000; fee-for-service insurance 2 million; public medical services 1·2 million; private doctors' clubs 100,000; and works clubs (including medical aid societies) about 3 million. On these estimates about 14 million individuals would have been covered by the above schemes. The remaining 13½ million or so would have paid private fees.

---

[1] *Ibid.*, rule 87.

[2] BMA, Medico-Political Committee, Documents 1936-37 MP75.

[3] RCNHI [1926], Appendices, p. 171.

[4] Ministry of Health, *Annual Report*, 1938-39.

[5] FSMA, *Annual Report*, 1945, in PRO MH77/94.

[6] RCNHI [1926], Q. 16,349.

[7] PRO MH77/93; NCFS, *Annual Reports*, 1930, 1938 1948.

TWO

The BMA's Dislike of Competition

The variety of sources of supply still in existence in the 1930s made it difficult for the BMA to maintain a cartel. Considerable pressures continued to prevent it from unilaterally fixing capitation rates. Even against the background of government price-fixing of national insurance rates and a professional policy of seeking increases up to government rates in the private contract sector, the profession lacked the power to get its way. This applied not only to contract practice; in insurance against medical fees, the BMA was unable to prevent doctors accepting, for instance, the two-thirds contribution of the National Deposit Friendly Society in full settlement of accounts. Wage limits to exclude higher-paid workers were not universally applied and, despite strong BMA pressure, consumer combinations which offered countervailing power to the organised profession survived.[1]

Market power of the medical institutes

Most notable among the organisations which offered competition and restrained medical fees were the friendly society medical institutes. In the 1930s the medical institutes had only about 150,000 voluntary members (in addition to national insurance members), but they were distributed throughout England in over 60 large towns. Only one serious competitor in a locality was required to upset BMA price-fixing, and the medical institutes consequently had an effect on prices out of all proportion to the size of their membership. This market power earned them the implacable hostility of the medical profession; as a result, when the NHS was being planned the BMA's hostility was decisive in ensuring that no role at all was permitted for medical institutes.

Throughout the life of the panel system, the BMA kept the Ministry of Health under constant pressure to discriminate against approved institutions. In March 1921, for instance, Alfred Cox

---

[1] For a full discussion of competition in the 1930s, Green [forthcoming].

wrote to the Ministry on behalf of the BMA complaining that the Norwich FSMI was charging 3s a quarter for juvenile members. The BMA felt this was too low and accused the Institute of subsidising juveniles out of their income from the national insurance scheme. Cox wrote again on 22 April emphasising that the BMA 'strongly objects' to the subsidisation of the non-insured. The Permanent Secretary (R. W. Harris) replied that he could not carry on the correspondence on an official footing but proposed a private chat when Cox was next in the Ministry. On 7 May Cox called in for his chat. An official note records the BMA's reasoning:

'From the BMA point of view it is particularly important that the assumption that these uninsured juveniles can be treated for the same charge as an insured person should not be established as a precedent which might be used in the event of the extension of GP treatment to the general population'.[1]

Medical institutes as 'embryo health centres'

By the time of the Royal Commission on National Health Insurance (RCNHI) of 1926, health centres formed an important part of the BMA's plans for health care; indeed, all progressive opinion was in favour of health centres, which offered larger possibilities for consultation between GPs and for the provision of improved diagnostic aids and specialist care. Ironically, the medical institutes, so mistrusted by the BMA and the Ministry of Health, were *health centres in embryo*, as at least one member of the Royal Commission had noted. But this made little difference to the generally hostile attitude adopted by the Royal Commission.[2] From the outset, the Royal Commission had shown little sympathy for medical institutes, as its questioning of the Independent Order of Rechabites fairly early in its proceedings indicates.[3]

The PEP report of 1937 also noticed that medical institutes were embryo health centres. It described two of the medical institutes it happened to stumble across as providing a comprehensive medical service 'which should be the model of any national system of medical services'. The two services were the Great Western Railway Medical Fund Society of Swindon, and the Llanelly and District Medical Service. The latter had 18,100 subscribers.[4] Established in 1847, the Great Western Railway Medical Fund Society at Swindon had, by 1944, 14 full-time

---

[1] PRO MH81/54.
[2] RCNHI [1926], Qs. 6,369-81.
[3] RCNHI [1926], Qs, 6,316-59.
[4] PEP [1937], pp. 151-2.

medical officers and consultants (plus visiting consultants), three full-time dental surgeons, and a 42-bed hospital with a large out-patient department. It catered for 40,205 people, around half the population of Swindon. Of these, 15,386 were covered by national insurance.[1]

Other medical institutes also continued to thrive until the NHS was founded. The Norwich FSMI had been founded in 1872, and by May 1944 it had four full-time medical officers, two qualified chemists, one dispenser and one assistant, in addition to clerical staff and a receptionist. The city was divided into four districts for home visits, each served by a particular doctor. When specialist consultations were required, the Institute paid 50 per cent of the fee. The Institute was managed by a committee, but 'clinical work was left to the clinician'.[2] As late as October 1947 it still had 13,746 members, of whom 9,161 were covered by national insurance. Hours of business at the Norwich FSMI were also far more attractive than those offered by many panel practitioners. In the 1930s the Institute was even open on Christmas Day and Good Friday between 9.30 and 10.00 a.m. for 'urgent' cases.[3]

In 1946, 22,800 people out of the town's total population of 24,000 were members of the Tredegar Workmen's Medical Aid Society. Miners and steelworkers contributed by pay-packet deductions of 2d in the £1, and other members 18s a year. The Society employed five doctors, one surgeon, two pharmacists, one masseuse (physiotherapist), a dentist and assistant, and a district nurse. For 4d a week free hospital treatment was also available. Spectacles could be obtained for 2s 6d and false teeth at less than cost price. Artificial limbs were free, as were injections, patent foods, drugs, wigs and X-rays. For those who had to go to hospital, a car was provided to the railway station and the first-class rail fare was paid. The doctors were paid according to the number of patients on their list, and usually earned about £380 a year. Private patients were allowed, but only about 5 per cent of the population remained outside the Society. It was managed by 30 delegates, who were mostly miners—the dreaded 'committee' of A. J. Cronin's *The Citadel*. Tredegar's was typical of other medical aid societies in South Wales.[4]

---

[1] PRO MH77/93.

[2] *Ibid.*

[3] PRO MH81/54.

[4] RCNHI [1926], Appendix XXXIX, para. 13.

THREE

The Demise of the Medical Institutes

During the Second World War there was much discussion of how primary medical care should be organised. One plan followed another in quick succession: the 'Brown Plan', the White Paper of 1944, the 'Willink Plan'. When the National Health Service Bill was passed in 1946, the NHS general practitioner service turned out to be very like the old 1911 panel system. The insurance committees were replaced by local executive councils. There was a degree of central control of the GP service through the Medical Practices Committee. Capitation payment was retained, and private practice was to continue, but the sale of practices was forbidden.

The wartime Coalition Government began planning a comprehensive medical service in February 1943, and in March Ernest Brown, Minister of Health, announced his proposals (the 'Brown Plan'). The South Wales and Monmouthshire Alliance of Medical Aid Societies (SWMA), worried about their future role under the Plan, asked to meet the Minister but was rebuffed. In December 1943 Henry Willink became Minister, and two months later published a White Paper, *A National Health Service*, which proposed to 'weld together' existing institutions. In March 1944 the Friendly Societies' Medical Alliance (FSMA) inquired how this 'welding' would be carried out, and subsequently a joint conference of the FSMA and the SWMA decided to ask the Minister why the White Paper did not refer to approved institutions. The Minister agreed to meet both organisations in April 1944 and subsequently Willink wrote to Sir Geoffrey Shakespeare, a sympathetic MP (for Norwich), that the medical institutes were not being overlooked: 'their valuable pioneering work is fully appreciated'.[1]

The friendly societies sought further meetings with the Minister throughout 1944. Civil servants advised him to decline to meet them until after the BMA's Representative Meeting in December. One senior adviser told Willink he suspected the alliances would

---

[1] PRO MH77/93.

merely ask 'that their existence should be preserved in the NHS . . . rather than submit helpful suggestions on the general form the GP service should take'. There was thus no real point in meeting them.

In December, civil servants finally advised that a meeting with the alliances *should* be held. One of them had scrawled on the back of a letter from the FSMA dated 11 December:

'I do not quite see how these people can be put off any longer. Indeed, I should have thought it was better now than later, since it is easier now to give a non-committal answer on the ground that there are still so many doubtful factors'.[1]

'Killing off' the competition

A civil service memorandum to the Minister dated 18 January 1945 advised:

'Their case is poor. They have always been disliked by the medical profession; they are not much thought of by the Department; and the Royal Commission of 1926 said they were "anomalous" '.[2]

Moreover, the Minister was told, their past advantage in providing a wider range of services than under the panel system would disappear under the new scheme. The Minister should therefore 'listen to their case and hold out no hopes, without finally announcing any decision to kill them'. In these circumstances it would be better to 'see them soon and get it over'. And a personal meeting with the Minister was thought advisable because of the interest in the matter displayed by Sir Geoffrey Shakespeare and because

'if we are in fact in the end going to kill them [they will] not then be able to complain that they have not been able to put their case in the highest quarters'.[3]

The alliances finally met the Minister in February 1945.

The medical institutes were never taken seriously by the Government and the Minister received a constant stream of advice from civil servants that they should be abandoned. The advice was invariably misleading and of a very low calibre. It was of the kind that flourishes because it is given in secret and cannot therefore be challenged publicly. There was no malice towards the friendly societies; they were simply seen as 'anomalous'. Above all, civil servants appear to have devoutly believed that the NHS would be a vast improvement on the *status quo*. They were by no means

---

[1] *Ibid.*   [2] *Ibid.*   [3] *Ibid.*

immune from the millennial expectations which sometimes seize whole populations at times of great stress and which on this occasion led to such advice as:

> 'But the societies cannot command the whole range of services which the patient is to be offered in the new scheme [.If] these services are not all at the societies' command, they cannot keep up with the standard elsewhere even if they are better at the start'.[1]

In other words, the medical institutes could not possibly be better than the planned NHS; and even if they were, they soon would not be. On the draft version of the above note to the Minister the contradiction had been spotted: the word 'better' had been ringed in pencil and a question mark placed in the margin. But it remained in the final version.

A proposal that the institutes could become agents for the Ministry of Health was strongly rejected. An agency agreement would mean:

> '. . . first, increased costs of administration, and secondly, the interposition of an extra link in the chain of responsibility—the doctor is responsible to the Society, which is responsible to the Health Service Authorities or the local 'insurance' committee, which are responsible to the patient's representatives, namely, Parliament. Any such extra link weakens the doctor's responsibilities to the patient and makes, e.g., complaints machinery more difficult to work, as has been found in practice'.[2]

It would also prevent 'so free a choice of doctor'. Moreover, the argument ran, the profession (the producer) was hostile to the institutes (the consumer), and to support them would therefore be to alienate the profession. It was also felt that to allow any 'contracting out' or 'other arrangements' would set a precedent such that before long groups like 'Christian Scientists and nature healers' would be demanding to be included.

Civil service ignorance

The memorandum which had been submitted to the Minister by the FSMA and the SWMA in February 1945 was answered point by point. The institutes observed that, because their medical officers consulted patients in the same premises, close co-operation and consultation were more easy. Apparently oblivious of his Department's espousal of health centres for this very reason, an official responded: 'Agreed, but a centralised service does not suit *all* patients, or all doctors'.

The institutes remarked that medical officers and dispensers

---

[1] *Ibid.* [2] *Ibid.*

could also co-operate more easily. The answer they received was that 'the general principle was that doctors should not dispense; centralised services are not the most convenient in all cases'. The official seemed unaware that medical institutes were not being proposed for all cases, and that medical institute doctors did not dispense.

The institutes further noted that their premises were purpose-built. The answer: 'Yes, but the premises are not always very good'. Premises did indeed vary, but they were among the best available anywhere.

The institutes also reminded the Government that they did not work for a profit. It is difficult to believe that the answer they received on this point was sincere: 'The fact that the Institutions do not work for profit should mean that there is no financial hardship if they are merged in the new service and lose their identity'. The provision of consultative and specialist services by the institutes was said to be 'good as far as it goes but the comprehensive service must go further'.

Finally, the alliances said that the approved institutions were prepared 'to co-operate in every way possible in order to maintain and improve the standard of service in the interests of the insured persons, wives and dependants'. The answer: 'This is gratifying but the scheme must be open to everyone who wants it, not merely insured persons, wives and dependants'. It seems the author of this passage was so overcome by millennial anticipation of the comprehensiveness of the NHS that he forgot that the expression 'insured persons, wives and dependants' was commonly taken to refer to every living soul!

False reassurance from the Government

At the February 1945 meeting, Willink rather disingenuously assured the FSMA and SWMA delegates that the Government's object was 'not unnecessarily to destroy existing institutions but to make the best use of the facilities they offered'.[1] The medical institutes were reassured. Nevertheless, at the General Election of July 1945, they contacted MPs in all areas where there was a medical institute to ask if they supported the preservation of approved institutions. The response was favourable, and the FSMA was surprised by the 'almost total unanimity' of the reactions.[2]

---

[1] Report of meeting issued by Ministry of Health, PRO MH77/94.

[2] FSMA, *Annual Report*, 1945, in PRO MH77/94.

The delegation which was received by the Minister in February 1945 had been accompanied by two MPs. One was Aneurin Bevan, who fully supported the SWMA at the meeting. In July he became Minister and began signing the same kinds of letters, drafted by the same officials, that Willink and Brown had signed before him. In September the SWMA asked to meet Bevan. He replied that it was 'too early'; he had not made up his mind how to proceed. In late October he put them off again. The following month the FSMA and the SWMA jointly approached the Minister for a meeting. Bevan declined once again, telling them that the 'general issues' were still under review. It was still too early. Finally, a meeting was agreed for January 1946.

Bevan began that meeting by admitting that he was 'somewhat embarrassed'. He was asked if he would like to see the alliance's statement in support of their case for continued existence. He replied:

'I know the valuable services rendered by Associations. I have been closely associated with them for many years, even from boyhood, so I cannot be told more than I already know, and it would therefore be a waste of your time and mine to go over the matter again. I will therefore outline to you the Government's Scheme'.[1]

Bevan presented the 10 delegates with an outline of the scheme. It was to be based 'primarily on health centres, a field in which the Medical Aid Societies had done valuable pioneering'. In the new health centres doctors were to be 'in consultation with each other'. Medical institute doctors 'would therefore be in isolation'. There was to be a distribution of doctors to areas in which they were most needed. 'How could we do that with your doctors?', Bevan asked. They were told that the scheme 'left no proper place for indirect agencies' like medical institutes. But they were assured that their experience would not be wasted and that there would be 'ample work' on the various committees concerned with administering the new scheme. But, Bevan added, there was no reason why the institutes could not provide benefits additional to the state scheme. A delegate pointed out that there would not be much scope for this in a 'full and comprehensive service'.

Bevan was again reminded of the comprehensive services available in Swindon and Tredegar. Were they now, a delegate asked, 'to be thrown on the scrap heap as redundant?' Bevan replied: 'I very much appreciate the splendid work you have done and are still doing. I am not emotional about Institutions but I am about people'. The Cabinet, he said, were 'determined not to have the

---

[1] *Ibid.*

scheme cluttered up by other agencies'. His conclusion was that:
'You have shown us the way and by your very efficiency you
have brought about your own cessation'.[1]

Three very closely related, but unspoken, notions seem to have
been at the root of the Government's thinking. The first was a
simple faith in the superiority of government provision over market
provision. Even though developments in the health-care market
outside the government scheme were considerable, and often
provided a model for reformers intent on forcing everyone into a
single government health scheme, freedom from government
interference continued to be poorly valued. By the 1930s, after
some years of government intervention, all improvements were
taken by 'progressive opinion' to be the result of the government
scheme and all problems the result of the continuing inadequacy
of the market-place or the unsatisfactory (but easily remediable)
nature of previous government intervention. Early mistakes were
not seen as inherent in government intervention as such, but
rather as arising from failures of personnel or programme. No
satisfactory effort was made to appraise the market as an alternative to intervention. If the market *was* compared, it was the market
before intervention—as if no change would have occurred with
or without government interference. Nor was there any recognition that government might have inadvertently stifled some
beneficial changes.

Enthusiasts for statism passionately believed that the new
scheme was going to be the best, and therefore to allow any other
kind of organisation to continue in being was pointless. It was
inconceivable that any alternative would be better. To permit non-
government agencies to continue would therefore be to complicate
matters to no purpose.

The 'synoptic delusion'

Closely allied to this simple faith in the superiority of government
was a second notion which Hayek has called the 'synoptic delusion'.[2] The notion is that a single person can hold in his mind
all the facts relevant to some social problem. The PEP report on
Britain's health services provides an example of the synoptic
delusion, and of its contradictory character:

'The mere fact that no comprehensive approach to the health services was
available and that it has taken a group of ordinarily intelligent people three

---

[1] FSMA, *Annual Report*, pp. 17-19, in PRO MH77/94.

[2] Hayek [1973], pp. 14-15.

years to hammer out this preliminary synthesis, is conclusive proof that the subject was in a serious state of confusion. The fact that the elementary information here given had to be collected by prolonged inquiry from so many different persons and agencies is itself a criticism for those who believe, as we do, that it is important to try to look at these services as a whole, and to judge how they are doing their job by examining them in relation to one another and to the needs they exist to satisfy. No one can be surprised if sectional and one-sided views are prevalent so long as the basis for a balanced and comprehensive view does not exist'.[1]

Having made this claim, the report proceeds to complain on the very next line that it is difficult to find a satisfactory answer to the question 'What are the health services?'. Its authors were, it seems, demanding a comprehensive view of a subject which they believed to be very complex and the boundaries of which they regarded as indistinct. It is tempting to conclude that one of the reasons they wanted a 'comprehensive system' was simply their frustration as professional researchers with the difficulties of investigating a complex subject. On several occasions the PEP report complains about the difficulty of gathering information about the non-state schemes. For example, referring to works clubs it says: 'Again, owing to the individual and *unorganised* nature of these insurances, it is impossible to ascertain the extent of provision'.[2] 'Unorganised' meant uncentralised, for plainly the schemes were organised in the ordinary sense.

The third notion was that change is not problematic. All thought was being directed to creating what was intended to be the best health service attainable. That some institutional structures are more amenable to progress than others was not on the agenda in 1945 and 1946. This example of the tendency of socialist thought to assume a static situation was identified by Ludwig von Mises.[3] Even though the pioneering work of the medical institutes was freely acknowledged, it appears to have been assumed that there would no longer be any need for pioneering institutions. The state scheme would take care of progress.

A letter to Anthony Eden's private secretary, written by Bevan's private secretary in April 1946 (no doubt with his approval), typifies the thinking of the day: 'We realise the splendid work' of the medical aid associations such as the Leamington Provident Dispensary. The reasons their services will no longer be necessary 'will be simply that provision by public organisation and from public funds will have caught up with pioneer voluntary effort in

---

[1] PEP [1937], p. 2.

[2] *Ibid.*, p. 150 (emphasis added).

[3] Von Mises [1981], p. 142 and p. 186.

that sphere'.[1] Without question, such a viewpoint minimally assumes that progress is unproblematic. It does not acknowledge that thought must be given to which of the institutional structures available to us most readily facilitates progress. And it shows no awareness that state socialism is very inferior to the market in facilitating progress.

Medical institute staff lose their livelihoods

The National Health Service Bill was published in March 1946, by which time the SWMA members had resigned themselves to their fate and were beginning to press for assurances that existing staff would be employed by the NHS. (The 51 medical institutes in England and Wales employed about 250 staff, around 100 of whom were full time.)

As an accidental outcome of the crushing of the medical institutes, around a dozen of their employees lost their livelihoods without compensation when the NHS came into being on 5 July 1948 and the institutes ceased to exist.

Fears that the NHS would be inferior

Evidence from Wales

The lay staff of the medical institutes were not the only 'accidental' casualties of the NHS. On 8 June 1948, with only four weeks to go before the NHS officially came into being, the SWMA brought information to Bevan's attention which appears to have alarmed him. It seemed that, in some areas, health-care provision was going to be worse after 5 July than before.

On 12 May 1948 an official of the Monmouthshire executive council had told the Welsh Board of Health that the new pharmaceutical service would be unsatisfactory in Tredegar. When the doctors of the Tredegar medical aid society, who carried out the dispensing, stopped doing so on 5 July—as the new scheme required—the two chemists' shops in the town 'could not . . . provide a service equal to the present'.[2] At the 8 June meeting, Bevan was reminded of this and other problems. He said he did not want the dispensing to go to the chemists' shops because 'in four or five years' time' health centres would be built and the dispensing would then have to go back to the health centres (a very optimistic belief as it turned out). He suggested that the

---

[1] PRO MH77/93.   [2] PRO MH77/94.

premises of the medical aid societies should be declared 'provisional health centres'.

In a note describing the Minister's feelings after that meeting, Bevan was said to be

> 'not at all satisfied that the Local Health Authorities in Monmouthshire and Glamorgan had taken adequate steps to ensure that the health facilities available after the 5th July would be at least as efficient as those available under the Medical Aid Societies'.[1]

And Bevan minuted his concerns for the benefit of Ministry staff. He emphasised two points: (i) the service provided after the appointed day must be at least as good as the day before; and (ii) where a medical aid society did not want its service to be taken over by a commercial chemist, it should be allowed to continue as a health centre, even if the building was not suitable. 'Anything could be designated a Health Centre', he insisted, and it could be improved later. On 9 June 1948 an instruction was issued embodying these principles.

Bevan's decision was never fully implemented, however. The premises at Tredegar, Ebbw Vale and Blaenavon were considered suitable for use as health centres and the remainder were not. At an angry meeting with the SWMA, officials of the Welsh Board of Health told the delegation that Bevan had originally intended to declare *all* the premises of the medical aid societies provisional health centres, but had eventually been prevailed upon by his officials not to do so.

On 1 July 1948, Bevan received a report from the Welsh Board of Health describing exactly what his revised decision would mean. The medical aid societies were carrying out dispensing from 19 centres in South Wales. They had two chemists and four dispensers, and the remaining dispensing was carried out by society doctors. The difficulty at Tredegar was resolved by taking over the premises as a health centre. In other areas doctors would be allowed to continue dispensing. Where commercial chemists were to take over, officials told Bevan that the new service would be satisfactory except in three places: Cwm (Ebbw Vale), Llwynpia (Mid-Rhondda) and Pontlottyn. Bevan was warned that his approval of the new arrangements could well mean 'trouble' in the Rhondda, although the position 'might be eased if it could be explained to the local people that a much better pharmaceutical service should result'. At Neath there was a 'small but excellent dispensary', but this would be displaced by a chemist's shop. At mid-Rhondda the dispenser was disabled. He was reported to have provided a

---

[1] *Ibid.*

good service for many years. (Nevertheless he eventually lost his job.)[1]

Why did Bevan reverse his promised decision? Officials appear to have feared bad publicity for the NHS. They told the SWMA on 4 July that they 'did *not* want to see press photographers publishing pictures of "provisional" health centres such as would be set up in Glamorgan' (emphasis in original). The Government, it seems, was trapped by its own rhetoric. The NHS was 'comprehensive', it was 'the best', and so *nothing*—however true it might be—could be allowed to contradict these claims. The premises of some of the medical aid societies were not as large as was felt desirable for a new NHS health centre. Thus it was better to have nothing, and even better to have an inferior service supplied by a commercial chemist, than to let the press claim the NHS was not 'the best'.

The spokesmen for the SWMA were said to be in a 'very angry mood' and officials felt the situation promised to become 'very ugly'. At one stage a 'general stoppage of work in the Rhondda' was threatened. On the appointed day the situation was officially described as 'extremely delicate'. The leaders of the local medical aid society were thought to be 'quite capable of engineering street corner meetings for the purpose of bringing about a breakdown of the NHS'—and had threatened to do so. As a result, the societies were allowed to continue functioning a little longer. By 6 July a meeting of all doctors in the Rhondda had been held. Most decided to conform. One doctor at Llwynpia who practised a mile from the nearest chemist decided to continue dispensing until a (planned) branch of Boots was opened. And Dr Williams of the Tonypandy central surgery told his patients to have their prescriptions dispensed by a chemist if they wished, or by the medical aid society dispenser, who was qualified as a dispenser but not as a pharmacist. The latter arrangement contravened the National Health Service Act.[2]

The standard retort to these findings from NHS partisans would doubtless be that they were 'only' teething problems. But the important issue is that there was no need to have created teething problems at all. The people of the Welsh valleys had created, and sustained and managed over many years, arrangements which suited them. It was within their power to improve those arrangements as they saw fit, as they had consistently done over many decades. The market *was* imperfect, but it was *constantly* being refined under pressure from consumers.

---

[1] *Ibid.*   [2] PRO MH77/94.

The experience described serves to illustrate a general truth about large-scale, comprehensive and compulsory social engineering: that the social engineers are irremediably ignorant. We may assume that Bevan's intentions towards the people of South Wales were benevolent. Yet he remained ignorant of the real effects the NHS was about to have (not only in South Wales generally but in his own constituency) until less than a month before the inauguration of the NHS. For a few days, after the facts were brought home to him, he acted decisively. Then he succumbed to the arguments of his officials.

The fate of the medical institutes in England

On the eve of the NHS in June 1948, there were 31 medical institutes in England. Of these, 17 were to be taken over by existing medical officers on 5 July; in four instances the county councils were planning to take them over to run as health centres; in one case, York, the future was uncertain; and in nine instances the buildings were no longer to be used by GPs.[1]

The four premises to be taken over by county councils to be run as health centres belonged to the former Luton FSMI, the Great Western Railway Medical Fund Society of Swindon, the Gloucester FSMA, and the Gloucester Provident Dispensary.[2]

The health centres, which were expected to be in the forefront of NHS primary care, took a long time to materialise. By 1959 only 10 had been built; and many of the 92 GPs using them did not do so as their main base.[3] In May 1966, after 18 years of the NHS, only 24 health centres had come into existence, although an additional 24 had been approved and were under construction.[4] Since then numbers have increased rapidly. Twenty years after the Act, however, *there were fewer health centres than there had been medical institutes before 1946.*

Conclusion

Before 1948 friendly society medical institutes and medical aid societies provided much-needed competition in the supply of medical care. This helped to contain prices in the non-panel sector. Perhaps more significant was the innovative role of medical

---

[1] *Ibid.*

[2] PRO MH77/95.

[3] *Parliamentary Debates*, House of Commons, 1959-60, vol. 615, cols. 11-12.

[4] *Parliamentary Debates*, House of Commons, 1966-67, vol. 728, col. 17.

institutes and medical aid societies. As Aneurin Bevan acknowledged, they had pioneered new services which it was hoped the NHS would make standard. Yet, under the illusion that the political process can provide for innovation as effectively as the market, all alternatives to the NHS monolith were excluded. Due partly to government efforts to satiate professional demands, but also to a misguided faith in the omniscience and organisational capacity of government, the final vestiges of competition in the supply of health care were driven out of existence.

List of References

Abel-Smith, B. [1976]: *Value For Money in Health Services*, London: Heinemann.

Acheson, H. W. K., and Henley, M. H. [1984]: *Clinical Knowledge and Education for General Practice*, Royal College of General Practitioners, Occasional Paper 27.

BMA [1984]: British Medical Association, *The Handbook of Medical Ethics*, London: BMA.

Berlant, J. L. [1975]: *Profession & Monopoly*, Berkeley: University of California Press.

Bosanquet, N. [1984]: 'How to save the nation's health: the social market view', *Economic Affairs*, vol. 4, no. 3, pp. 49-50.

Burke, E. [1907]: *The Works of Edmund Burke*, (6 vols.) London: Oxford University Press/The World's Classics.

Culyer, A. J. [1976]: *Need and the National Health Service*, London: Martin Robertson.

Culyer, A. J. [1982]: 'The NHS and the market: images and realities', in McLachlan, G., and Maynard, A., *The Public/Private Mix for Health*, London: Nuffield Provincial Hospitals Trust, pp. 23-55.

Detsky, A. S. [1978]: *The Economic Foundations of National Health Policy*, Cambridge, Mass.: Ballinger.

Eaton, G., and Parish, P. [1976]: 'Sources of drug information used by general practitioners', *Journal of the Royal College of General Practitioners*, vol. 26, supplement, no. 1.

Enthoven, A. C. [1978]: 'Consumer-choice health plan' (first of two parts), *New England Journal of Medicine*, vol. 298, no. 12, pp. 650-58.

Enthoven, A. C. [1978]: 'Consumer-choice health plan' (second of two parts), *NEJM*, vol. 298, no. 13, pp. 709-20.

Evan, R. G. [1974]: 'Supplier-induced demand: some empirical evidence and implications', in Perlman, M. (ed.), *The Economics of Health and Medical Care*, New York: Wiley, pp. 162-73.

Feldstein, M. S. [1967]: *Economic Analysis for Health Service Efficiency: Econometric Studies of the British National Health Service*, Amsterdam: North Holland.

Friedman, M. [1962]: *Capitalism and Freedom*, Chicago: University of Chicago Press.

Friedman, M. & R. [1980]: *Free to Choose*, London: Macmillan.

Fuchs, V. R. [1978]: 'The supply of surgeons and the demand for operations', *Journal of Human Resources,* vol. 13, Supplement, pp. 35-36.

GMC [1983]: General Medical Council, *Professional Conduct & Discipline: Fitness to Practise*, London: GMC, August.

Green, D. G. [1982]: *The Welfare State: For Rich or For Poor?*, IEA Occasional Paper 63, London: Institute of Economic Affairs.

Green, D. G. [1984]: 'Doctors versus workers', *Economic Affairs*, Supplement, vol. 5, no. 1, pp. i-xii.

Green, D. G. [Forthcoming]: *Working Class Patients and the Medical Establishment*, London: Temple Smith.

Hadley, J., Holahan, J., and Scanlon, W. [1979]: 'Can fee-for-service reimbursement co-exist with demand creation?', *Inquiry*, vol. 16, pp. 247-58.

Hayek, F. A. [1968]: *The Confusion of Language in Political Thought*, Occasional Paper 20, London: IEA.

Hayek, F. A. [1973]: *Law, Legislation and Liberty*: vol. I, *Rules and Order*, pp. 14-15. London: Routledge and Kegan Paul.

Hayek, F. A. [1978]: 'Competition as a discovery procedure', in *New Studies in Philosophy, Politics, Economics, and the History of Ideas*, pp. 179-90. London: Routledge & Kegan Paul.

Huxley, T. H. [1884]: 'The state and the medical profession', *Nineteenth Century*, vol. 15, pp. 230-1.

ICM [1984]: Institute for Complementary Medicine, *Report on Trends in Complementary Medicine* (September).

Jones, P. R. [1980]: 'The growth of the British Medical Association', in Leaper, R. A. B. (ed.), *Health, Wealth and Housing*, Oxford: Blackwell/Martin Robertson, pp. 177-202.

Kessel, R. A. [1958]: 'Price discrimination in medicine', *Journal of Law & Economics*, vol. 1, pp. 20-53.

Klein, R. [1982]: Private practice & public policy: regulating the frontiers', in McLachlan, G. and Maynard, A. [1982].

Le Grand, J., and Robinson, R. [1976]: *The Economics of Social Problems*, London: Macmillan.

McLachlan, G., and Maynard, A. (eds.) [1982]: *The Public/Private Mix For Health*, London: Nuffield Provincial Hospitals Trust.

Macaulay, T. B. [1967]: *History of England*, (4 vols.), London: Heron Books.

Marrinker, M. [1984]: 'Developments in primary care', in Teeling-Smith, G. (ed.), *A New NHS Act for 1996?*, London: Office of Health Economics.

Maynard, A. [1980]: 'How not to regulate the medical profession', in Leaper, R. A. B. (ed.), *Health, Wealth and Housing*, Oxford: Blackwell/Martin Robertson, pp. 139-58.

Maynard, A. [1982]: 'The regulation of public and private health care markets', in McLachlan, G., and Maynard, A. (eds.) [1982], pp. 471-512.

Maynard, A., & Ludbrook, A. [1980]: 'What's wrong with the National Health Service?', *Lloyds Bank Review*, October, pp. 27-41.

Maynard, A., and Williams, A. [1984]: 'Privatisation and the National Health Service', in Le Grand, J., and Robinson, R. (eds.), *Privatisation and the Welfare State*, London: George Allen & Unwin.

Merrison [1975]: *Report of the Committee of Inquiry into the Regulation of the Medical Profession* (chairman: A. W. Merrison), Cmnd. 6018, London: HMSO.

Mill, J. S. [1861]: *Considerations on Representative Government*, Everyman edn. 1972 (published with *On Liberty & Utilitarianism*) London: J. M. Dent.

Monopolies Commission [1970]: *A report on the general effect on the public interest of certain restrictive practices so far as they prevail in relation to the supply of professional services*, Cmnd. 4463, London: HMSO.

Newhouse, J. P. [1981]: 'The demand for medical care services: a retrospect and a prospect', in van der Gaag, J., and Perlman,

M. (eds.), *Health, Economics, and Health Economics*, Amsterdam: North Holland.

Newhouse, J. P. *et al.* [1982]: *Some Interim Results from a Controlled Trial of Cost Sharing in Health Insurance*, Santa Monica, California: Rand Corporation, R-2847-HHS.

Newhouse, J. P., Williams, A. P., *et al.* [1979]: *The Geographic Distribution of Physicians: Is the Conventional Wisdom Correct?*, Paper presented at the American Economic Association meetings, Atlanta, Georgia.

OHE [1977]: Office of Health Economics, *Sources of Information for Prescribing Doctors in Britain*, London: OHE.

PEP [1937]: *Report on the British Health Services*, London: Political and Economic Planning.

PMSUP [1910]: *Report as to the Practice of Medicine and Surgery by Unqualified Persons in the United Kingdom*, Cd. 5422, London: HMSO.

Popper, K. [1961]: *The Poverty of Historicism*, 2nd edn., with corrections. London: Routledge & Kegan Paul.

RCNHI [1926]: *Royal Commission on National Health Insurance: Report*, Cmd. 2596, London: HMSO.

RCNHS [1979]: *Royal Commission on the National Health Service: Report*, Cmnd. 7615, London: HMSO.

Sloan, F. A., and Feldman, R. [1978]: 'Competition among physicians', in Greenberg, W. (ed.), *Competition in the Health Care Sector: Past, Present, and Future*, Proceedings of a conference sponsored by the Bureau of Economics, Federal Trade Commission.

Smith, A. [1776]: *The Wealth of Nations*, Everyman edn. 1977, London: J. M. Dent.

Stevens, R. B., and Yamey, B. S. [1965]: *The Restrictive Practices Court: A Study of the Judicial Process and Economic Policy*, London: Weidenfeld and Nicolson.

Titmuss, R. M. [1959]: 'Health', in Ginsberg, M. (ed.), *Law and Opinion in England in the 20th Century*, London: Stevens and Sons.

Tullock, G. [1976]: *The Vote Motive*, Hobart Paperback No. 9, London: Institute of Economic Affairs.

Abbreviations

BMA   British Medical Association

BMJ   *British Medical Journal*

FSMA   Friendly Societies' Medical Alliance

GMC   General Medical Council

NCFS   National Conference of Friendly Societies

NDFS   National Deposit Friendly Society

NHS   National Health Service

PRO   Public Record Office

RFS   Registrar of Friendly Societies

SWMA   South Wales and Monmouthshire Alliance (of Medical Aid Societies)

Some recent IEA publications

Hobart Paperback 20

Farming for Farmers?
A critique of agricultural support policy

Richard Howarth 1985 xvi + 144 pp. £4·00

'Richard Howarth argues with a wealth of supporting evidence that the withering away of the Common Agricultural Policy would not only serve the interests of consumers, but also do no great harm to the majority of producers.' J. Bruce-Gardyne, *Sunday Telegraph*

'Mr Howarth shows a grasp of the real world of farming and the Common Agriculture Policy. His suggestion that the CAP should be allowed, and encouraged, to continue the withering-away process and his ideas on the equivalent of redundancy payments for miners or steelworkers are . . . well thought out.' *Big Farm Weekly*

Occasional Paper 71

No, Minister!
A radical challenge on economic and social policies from speeches in the House of Lords

Ralph Harris 1985 £1·80

'. . . debates a measure in Britain's House of Lords calling for more equality.' *Wall Street Journal* (Brussels)

Occasional Paper 72

Wage-Fixing Revisited
A revised and expanded text of the fourth Robbins Lecture

J. E. Meade 1985 £1·50

'The Institute of Economic Affairs has chosen a timely moment to publish Professor James Meade's paper . . . Professor Meade, winner of the Nobel prize for economics in 1977 and one of the authors of the 1944 White Paper on employment policy addresses a familiar theme. Wage determination is the central problem facing democratic economies and, without a radical change in the system of wage-fixing in Britain, the alleviation of unemployment will only be achieved at the expense of far higher inflation.'

The Times, in an Editorial

Research Monograph 39

Competition and Home Medicines

W. Duncan Reekie and **Hans G. Ötzbrugger**   1985   £1·80

'It deserves a read, and—so far as I am aware—the OFT has left the retail chemists well alone hitherto. From what Messrs Reekie and Ötzbrugger have to tell us, this is perhaps an omission.

'Put simply, their thesis is that, if Norman Fowler wants to save some more money for the NHS . . . then, instead of stamping on the fingers of the drugs firms, he could try loosening up on self-prescribing . . .

'I can't readily imagine Norman Fowler taking on this hornet's nest unprompted. But if the OFT were first to call in question whether the present rather cosy rules for chemists are necessarily in the true interests of consumers, that might be a different matter.'   Jock Bruce-Gardyne, *Sunday Telegraph*

Hobart Paper 102

Whose Business?

Brian Griffiths and **Hugh Murray**   1985   £2·50

'What price business schools, and who should pay it? The question is causing anxiety among the 900 academic staff of Britain's 27 colleges and university departments running full-time courses for Masters degrees in Business Administration.

'Since the MBA courses have several times been the main target of complaint about unduly academic approaches to teaching management, the schools are no strangers to criticism. But never before has the criticism led to a public proposal that they should be shorn of their state grants, on grounds that the need to pay their own way would make them concentrate less on scholarly pursuits and more on helping working managers to improve their practical skills.

'The challenge is sharpened by coming from inside the management teaching profession: from Professors Brian Griffiths and Hugh Murray of the City University Business School in London who set out their arguments in a report published by the IEA . . .'
                    Michael Dixon, *Financial Times*

'It is a symptom of our times that anything published by the Institute of Economic Affairs receives wide, even rapt, attention. . . . [But] not all IEA publications deserve the uncritical admiration which they receive. Certainly *Whose Business?* by two City University business school professors . . . need not be taken too seriously. . . . The authors seem to forget that "markets" can be levellers as well as leaders.'
                    The Times Higher Education Supplement, in an Editorial